Table of Contents

Chapter 1: Assess Needs, Assets, and Capacity for Health Education

Assessing needs, assets and capacities for health education requires planning, implementing, and evaluating programs for a given setting or an at-risk population. The main purpose of a needs assessment is to identify the attitudes, beliefs, and knowledge that contribute to the behaviors of individuals or groups in a community or certain setting. By completing all of the above, a health educator can specifically identify the needs of a population, community, or individual in order of importance and prioritize the most and least important changes to be made. Once all health problems and issues have been identified, a health educator can create the most beneficial program for all involved.

In this chapter, through a needs assessment, you will learn the importance of assessing needs, assets, and capacities by identifying all factors related to the current health status of the target population. Additionally, data from various government resources and data collected through various formats available will be used. Developing a program that addresses attitudes, beliefs, and knowledge will allow each individual to make better decisions about his/her health. The following are terms, concepts, and methods to assess needs, assets, and capacities in the health education field.

Community Capacity Inventory
A Community Capacity Inventory is an asset or community resource used to improve the quality of life in the community. It can be a person like a church member who organizes a discussion on spirituality or a firefighter who teaches CPR or other safety classes. Community assets can also be a physical structure like a church, library, school, hospital, or recreation center. It might also be a public place that belongs to the community like a park or other open area. Other assets are community services that make life more convenient like early childhood education centers or public transportation. It might also be a business that provides local jobs that support the local economy. Everyone in the community has the potential to be an asset with their skills and talents that can support health education efforts in the community.

Reliability
Reliability determines how consistently a measurement of knowledge or skill produces similar results under various conditions. If a measurement is highly reliable, it will yield consistent results over time. There are four ways to estimate a measurement's reliability:

1. Inter-observer:
   This is determined by how many different evaluators or observers examine the same presentation, project, paper, demonstration, or performance and agree on its overall rating.

2. Test-retest:
   This is determined by how often the same performance or test items evaluated at two different times yield similar results.

3. Parallel-forms:
   These are determined by examining how often two different measurements of skill or knowledge yield similar results.

4. Split-Half Reliability:
   This is determined by comparing half of a set of tests with another half and identifying how often they yield comparable results.

Validity

Validity is how often an instrument accurately measures what it's intended to measure. Over time, if an instrument is unreliable and returns erratic results, it cannot be considered valid. In other words, an instrument must be reliable to be considered valid. Rater Reliability is determined using consistent methods to rate a test, sample, or measurement.

Content validity guarantees that an overall sample of the content being measured is represented properly. The identified content must be accurately represented by the test items with a panel or group of experts used for testing validity.

Criterion validity directly considers the accuracy of a measure by comparing a selected measure with another valid measure.

Predictive validity forecasts or recognizes an association between the identified concept or form and something else. It is common to conduct one measurement at an earlier time and use it to predict a later measurement.

Concurrent validity exists when the identified measurement positively relates with a previous, valid measurement. The measurements can be associated with similar or different forms or concepts.

Construct validity ensures that the assessment measures the form or concept it claims to measure. Proof or presentation of comparative test performance results or pre- or post-testing of concept implementation can determine construct validity.

Discriminant validity identifies or illustrates that the measures that should not be related. The lack of correlation establishes discriminant validity.

Variables

Continuous Data

Maintaining a computerized data system is important for continually gathering, reviewing, and reporting program information. For example, program administers, policymakers, families, and investors will need this data to determine how services and resources are being used. A continuous data system should include the following:

- Demographic information
- Concerns and issues
- Actions taken
- Outcomes of each case

Discrete Data

New technology analyzes and tracks discrete data elements from narrative, transcribed reports. This process is accomplished by writing queries and comparing them to report databases concurrent with a review of 'man hours' and replaced with discrete data from narrations or speech-generated documents. Queries can be designed to pinpoint specific data elements across an entire population. The data is used to compile detailed reports that lighten the workload for case reviewers and ensure quality measurements with clinical documentation. Discrete data from narrations can be used to:

- Create patient or student action lists
- Add to electronic health records
- Target specific areas that need improvement
- Accurately chart reviews so only failed cases meeting query criteria are reviewed

Purpose Statement

The goal of health education is to optimize the health and wellness of individuals, groups, and communities with programs and services that empower and create awareness through presentations, outreach events, and other forms of communication. Some of the key topics addressed are health, fitness, nutrition, stress/time management, smoking, alcohol, and drug abuse. Programs are designed to help change behaviors both individually and environmentally.

Detailed Documentation

Detailed documentation of all cases and programs is required in health education. All reports and documents, such as exam reports, referral letters, and other important forms become part of legal records. They serve as a foundation for ongoing decision-making, maximized reimbursement, and risk management of all resources. Healthcare documentation specialists need extensive knowledge of anatomy, medical terminology, physiology, medical procedures, pharmacology, and other medical terms. Clinical knowledge is important for interpreting and understanding all situations in health education, especially constantly evolving new technologies and expansive medical language. Many doctors rely on healthcare document specialists to ensure their medical reports are complete and accurate. Some healthcare providers rely on voice recognition software to help complete documentation accurately; however, further editing is always required. It's important to keep nearby reference materials, such as medical dictionaries, diagnostic guides, coding manuals, and procedural guides. Accuracy is key, and medical records are confidential. Since most reports are sent by email, security and back-up storage, as well as virus protection, are extremely important.

Search Strategies
Educational and information strategies focus on delivering information designed to increase knowledge and awareness as a prerequisite for behavioral change. General health information can include material about chronic disease and reducing risk, weight loss and maintenance, nutrition, and physical activity. Of course, these strategies do not include any policy or environmental strategies.

Systematic Reviews
Systematic reviews are designed to improve the cultural competence of health education professionals. Data is gathered before and after evaluations to compare and grade evidence as poor, fair, good, or excellent using predetermined criteria. There is excellent evidence that cultural competence training improves:
- Knowledge of health education professionals
- Attitudes and skills of health professionals
- Patient and student satisfaction

Cultural competence training is emerging as a strategy for improving the knowledge, attitudes, and skills of health professionals. However, evidence that it improves patient adherence to therapy, health outcomes, and equity of services across racial and ethnic groups is still lacking. Future research should focus on these outcomes and determine which teaching methods and content are most effective.

Mixed Methods
Mixed Methods research is defined as a research approach or methodology focusing on research questions requiring real-life understanding and perspective based on cultural influences. Using multiple methods, such as in-depth interviews or intervention trials, highlights the strengths of each one and frames them within philosophical and theoretical positions. Researchers using mixed methods often create and use explicit, diverse philosophical positions that bridge worldviews and practical perspectives. However, many find the mixed method research too challenging because of tensions created by different beliefs. However, it can also be an opportunity to transform these tensions into new knowledge using diverse approaches and signifying the research question or problem. Transformation creates a more democratic society or framework that permeates the entire research process and use of results. Mixed method studies provide opportunities for the integration of a variety of perspectives and theories, yielding strong qualitative research focusing on the meaning of human life and experience.

Approach
The best approach for mixed methods research is to yield efficient data collection procedures and facilitate group comparison within communities. Typical approaches include surveys; observation studies; case-controlled studies; random, controlled trials; and time-series designs. Mixed methods research begins with the assumption that

investigators understand social and health worlds and are able to gather evidence based on questions and theories. Social inquiry targets various sources that influence a given problem like policies, families, organizations, or individuals. Quantitative methods are ideal for measuring occurrences of known phenomenon. Qualitative methods identify previously unknown processes, explanations of how and why phenomena occur (including the span of their effects). Gathering evidence involves collecting both quantitative and qualitative data and combining the strength of both to answer all research questions.

Propriety

Propriety and feasibility standards are designed to consider policies, resources, and administrative and legislation factors. The optimal standard for community-based health promotion depends on the setting and circumstances of each situation. This approach creates a situation where both funders and policymakers support evaluation designs that fit the community.

Accuracy

Increasing the accuracy of people's self-perceptions of physical activity is important to consider when incorporating strategies for promoting physical activity in consistently inactive populations.

Feasibility

The feasibility of procedures to assess a workplace, group, individual, or community evaluates risks and needs of hazard reduction depending on the situation, workplace, and environment.

Utility

Utility regulation focuses on protecting consumers from abuse by firms with substantial market power, supporting investment by protecting investors from arbitrary government action, and promoting economic efficiency. While competition can reduce the need for regulation in utility industries, most industries contain monopolies where the benefits of regulation potentially outweigh the costs. Regulating utilities is complicated because prices for utility services are usually politically motivated. There are no votes to raise utility prices, and history is replete with examples of justifiable price increases being withheld at investors' expense and consumers' long-term interests.

Investors are aware of these pressures and the vulnerability of their usually large, long-term, and immobile investments. Unless a government has credibly committed to rules and regulations that ensure an opportunity to earn reasonable returns, private investment will not occur. Weak credibility will be reflected in higher capital costs and tariffs. In privatization, this situation translates into smaller gains from sales of existing enterprises and higher financing costs for new projects.

The long-term nature of most infrastructure investments makes creating credible commitments difficult. Highly specific rules can assure investors and lower capital costs, but they also make it difficult to adjust regulation to unforeseen developments, including changes in technology and market conditions. They also make it difficult to tailor responses to situations and provide incentives for efficiency. There is an important tradeoff between reducing the risk of expropriation, and with it capital costs, and retaining the flexibility to pursue efficiency and other objectives.

When designing regulatory systems, then, policymakers must resolve two fundamental challenges: how much discretion regulatory systems contain and how that discretion should be managed to reduce the risk of misuse and capital costs.

Utilization-focused Inputs/Outputs

Funding through in-kind donations, office space, and buildings for family resource centers must be allocated based on needs/asset assessments that will improve practices and on changed policies that are modified by increased inputs. Using outputs that include knowledge, increased skills, and changed attitudes and behaviors improve systems and, ultimately, the outcome. For example, funding for childcare provider training suggests centralizing immunization records to coordinate with parent education delivery system produces the ultimate outcome.

Outcomes

Short-term Outcomes

The short-term effects of a health education program can be measured through interactive meetings, educational brochures, informational websites, and a consultation with a health educator. Short-term outcomes focus on the needs of the patients, groups, and individuals in need of information. An educational program that positively influences the behavior of those involved is considered a short-term outcome.

Intermediate Outcomes

The evaluation of intermediate outcomes involves case managers, program directors, local evaluators, workers, and stakeholders that review their local health system action plan, which includes staff perceptions of all program components. Community issues, project design, and implementation all affect intermediate outcomes. Outreach, case management, and health education all contribute to perceived achievements of intermediate outcomes.

Long-term Outcomes

In long-term outcomes, health returns and education outweigh financial returns simply because people value health. Education increases life expectancy, and understanding how education affects health is important for long-term outcomes.

Evaluations

Health education evaluations ensure program success. There are various types of evaluations that incorporate tools for initiating programs. They include:

Formative Evaluation

Formative evaluations provide information needed to adjust teaching and learning during the/an ongoing process. It allows students to measure their understanding during the learning process. The formative evaluation process guides teacher decisions about future instruction and programs. Some examples include:

- Observations
- Asking questions
- Initiating discussions
- Graphic organizers
- Self-assessments
- Visual representations
- Whiteboards
- Quizzes

Process Evaluation

Process evaluation is used to document and monitor program implementation, which helps health educators understand the relationship between specific program factors and outcomes. Process evaluation has become more complex because more people recognize its importance and utility. There are some models and frameworks available to health educators to help develop a comprehensive process-evaluation plan for targeted programs. Suggested components for a process-evaluation plan include reliability, reach, recruitment, and context.

Summative Evaluation

A summative evaluation defines all viable solutions to a problem or issue and facilitates health education program implementation. The focus and sophistication of evaluation designs vary among education programs; however, they are used both during and after a program. Presented data illustrates the utility of a summative evaluation model when applied to a realistic test situation, yielding many advantages including financial issues and content.

Impact Evaluation

Impact evaluation assesses the immediate effect of a program on the behaviors of program participants. The types of information gathered include:

- Increased knowledge
- Behavioral changes
- Improved disease management
- Lifestyle changes

The goal is to assess whether the program activities produced the outcomes identified in that program's objectives. In the case of a nutrition education program, impact evaluation examines program participants' increases in healthy eating practices; increases in knowledge of healthy eating practices; and changes in health indicators like weight, cholesterol, and blood pressure.

Pretests and Post-Tests

Pretests and post-tests are often used to provide evidence of increased participant knowledge. A pretest is conducted before a program to gauge program participant knowledge before program activity implementation. A post-test is identical to the pretest, but is conducted after the program has concluded. By comparing the results of the two tests, planners can identify increases in program participant knowledge.

Outcome Evaluation

Outcome evaluation assesses a program's effects on the ultimate objectives including changes in social benefits, health, and quality of life. Information gathered in an outcome evaluation determines whether a program is impacting life quality and health status. Is it helping reduce chronic disease? Is it improving eating habits? Is weight loss occurring? Is exercise becoming habitual?

An outcome evaluation is conducted months after a program has been completed to determine if the program had the intended impact. Attitudes, behaviors, and knowledge of program participants can be surveyed to determine if the participants retained their health improvements and knowledge after the program ended.

Program Evaluation Questions

Five Critical Elements for Ensuring Evaluation Use

Evaluating a program requires a systematic method for collecting, analyzing, and using the gathered information to answer questions about each project, program, and policy.

1. Is the program efficient and effective? In both private and public sectors, investors and stakeholders will want to know if the programs they are funding, voting for, and implementing are achieving the intended effect based on the costs involved.
2. How can the program be improved? Is it worthwhile? Improving programs by offering alternatives for achieving program goals must be addressed.
3. Who can help answer these questions? Evaluators must answer these questions, which should be discussed by both the stakeholders and evaluators.
4. What are the qualitative and quantitative methods used in program research?
5. What backgrounds do program evaluators have? Do they have a sociology, psychology, social work, or economics background?

Dissemination

Dissemination determines what you are trying to achieve by performing it through distribution, broadcasting, or spreading information. Consider dissemination in the following ways:

1. Creating Awareness of your project is useful and recognized by your target audience through detailed knowledge of the work done through activities and outcomes. Creating this awareness can help build a profile and identity within the community.

16

2. Creating Understanding of your project and work will benefit targeted groups and individuals.
3. Dissemination for Action refers to a changed training or practice that results from adopting materials, products, and approaches offered by your project. To effect real change, groups and individuals must possess the correct skills and knowledge to understand the work required to achieve goals.

Logic Model

A 'logic model' visualizes how a program or project will work, including the theories and assumptions that highlight the expected work and activities necessary to achieve desired outcomes. Most commonly employed in program planning and evaluation, they identify conceptual and operational elements associated with intended outcomes.

Evaluation Model

An evaluation model assesses the quality of evaluation activities to determine whether they are well-designed and working optimally. Standards are recommended as criteria for judging the quality of a program's efforts in health education.

Centers for Disease Control (CDC) Six-Step Framework

The CDC's Framework for Program Evaluation in Health education is a guide to effectively evaluate public health programs and use the findings to improve programs and decision-making. While the framework is described in steps, the actions are not always clearly defined and are often completed in a cyclical, back-and-forth effort. Developing an evaluation plan is an ongoing process. During the process, you may need to revisit a step and/or complete discrete steps concurrently. Within each step of the framework, there are important components to consider. The steps include:
1. Engaging stakeholders
2. Describing the program
3. Focusing the evaluation design
4. Gathering credible evidence
5. Justifying conclusions
6. Ensuring use and sharing learned lessons

Additionally, the following evaluation standards will enhance evaluation quality by guarding and protecting against potential mistakes.
- **Utility standards** ensure an evaluation will serve the information needs of the intended users.
- **Feasibility standards** ensure an evaluation will be realistic, prudent, diplomatic, and frugal.
- **Propriety standards** ensure an evaluation will be conducted legally, ethically, and with regard for the welfare of those involved in the evaluation and those affected by its results.
- **Accuracy standards** ensure an evaluation will reveal and convey technically adequate information about the features that determine the worth or merit of the evaluated program.

Attainment

Community partnerships participate in many activities that are related and occur at similar times. The model components are interrelated and may require action plan refinement to guide community action and change, according to participant needs and goals, through changes in policy, public funding, or other means. The capacity for change relates to your mission and can affect outcomes. Other departments or communities addressing similar concerns may emulate your successful initiatives.

Some communities have some freedom in deciding what to do, while other partnerships may require more "tried-and-true" strategies requested by stakeholders. This approach is accomplished by implementing the same program strategies, but enhancing them by adding a catalyst for change to help achieve the desired outcome. Adapting involvements to fit community needs creates an approach that "belongs" to the participants and is something to be proud of and will likely remain in the program. This increases their ability to solve their specific problems. In their efforts to create a comprehensive community initiative, leaders must know what does and doesn't work.

Framework for Program Evaluation

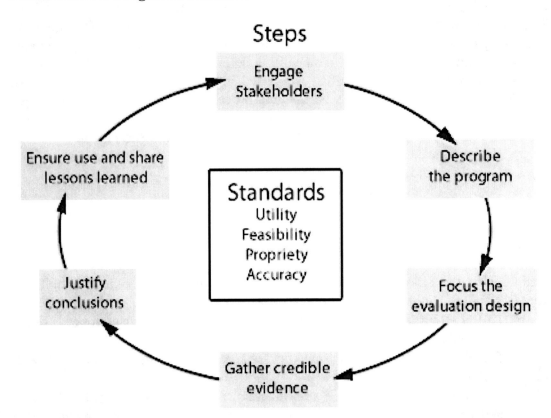

Six connected steps can be used as a starting point to modify an evaluation for a particular public health effort at a particular time. An order exists for fulfilling each step – generally, the earlier steps provide the foundation for subsequent progress.

1. **Engage stakeholders**, including those involved in program operations and those served or affected by the program, and primary evaluation users.

18

2. **Describe the program** including the need; expected effects; activities; resources; and stage, context, and logic models.
3. **Focus the evaluation design** to assess the most-concerning issues to stakeholders while using time and resources as efficiently as possible. Consider the purpose, users, uses, questions, methods, and agreements.
4. **Gather credible evidence** to strengthen evaluation judgments and following recommendations. These aspects of evidence gathering typically affect perceptions of credibility: indicators, sources, quality, quantity, and logistics.
5. **Justify conclusions** by linking them to gathered evidence and judging them against values or standards set by stakeholders. Justify conclusions on evidential basis using these five elements: standards, analysis/synthesis, interpretation, judgment, and recommendations.
6. **Ensure use and share learned lessons using** these steps: design, preparation, feedback, follow-up, and dissemination.

There are many options and potential levels of detail to a logic model, countless potential stakeholders, and a large number of potential ways to gather evidence. The Framework asks you to apply each of the 4 groups of evaluation standards as a "lens" to help identify the best approaches at each step.

Effective program evaluation is a systematic way to improve and consider public health actions. Evaluation involves useful, feasible, ethical, and accurate procedures. The term "*program*" is used in the framework to describe any organized public health action. Programs can include:
- Direct service interventions
- Community mobilization efforts
- Research initiatives
- Surveillance systems
- Policy development activities
- Outbreak investigations
- Laboratory diagnostics
- Communication campaigns
- Infrastructure building projects
- Training and education services
- Administrative systems

Health Behaviors

Factors that Influence Health Behaviors
The range of personal, social, economic, and environmental factors that influence health are known as *determinants of health*. Determinants of health are separated into several broad categories:
- Policymaking
- Social factors
- Health services

19

- Individual behavior
- Biology and genetics

It is the interrelationships among these factors that determine individual and population health. Because these interventions target multiple determinants of health, they are most likely to be effective. Determinants of health reach beyond the boundaries of traditional healthcare, and public health sectors, such as education, housing, transportation, agriculture, and environment, can be important allies in improving population health.

Behavioral Factors

Behavior is influenced by individual attributes as well as by living conditions. Altering policies, practices, and life conditions can directly and indirectly influence individual behavior. Behavioral factors effect change in individual behaviors. Interventions that target identified factors create conditions that not only reduce high-risk behavior, but also prevent adopting them. Structural interventions are important and underused approaches for improving our nation's health.

Environmental Factors

There is a growing recognition of the environmental role in influencing general and behavioral health. For example, the obesity epidemic continues to be brought into the mainstream, highlighting the importance of environment including obesity-risk behaviors that require a change in environment. Essentially, obesity is a product of our environment, like consumption of supersized soft drinks, sedentary behaviors at home in front of the computer or television, and the lack of exercise among adults. The study of environmental factors influencing our nutrition and physical activity is still considered a new science, but continues to gain momentum.

Individual Factors

Physical activity is influenced on an individual level, based on the availability of exercise equipment, for example. Strategies to change health behaviors have focused on individual factors such as skills, knowledge, and beliefs. Shaping individual health behavior can be challenging, but it is influenced by environment.

Enabling Factors

Enabling factors are part of the model for planning and promoting community health and evaluations, and they provide a guide to assessing health and quality-of-life needs of individuals and populations. They include planning, implementing, and evaluating strategies and programs designed to meet those needs, which involves a process of designing effective strategies to address behaviors that lead to health problems. Predisposition is one factor; however, community enabling resources, such as health facility availability, and personal enabling resources, such as people, know how to access and use the offered services.

Enabling factors make it possible or easier for individuals or groups to change their behavior or environment. Enabling factors include:
- Resources
- Living conditions
- Societal support
- Skills that facilitate healthy behavior

Predisposing Factors
Predisposing factors are present in individuals with a family history of a disease or health issue, such as diabetes or heart disease, and are aware of the risks. For example, diabetes majorly contributes to mortality and generates both direct and indirect costs. The prevalence of diabetes among adults in the U.S. has increased substantially, plus it is estimated that 35-50% of people with type II diabetes have not been diagnosed. As a result, at the time of their diagnosis, many people must deal with early complications of the disease. Knowledge of a predisposition to the disease can significantly affect prevention and reversal.

Reinforcement Factors
There are neighborhoods throughout the U.S. that are considered disadvantaged or unhealthy and reinforce unhealthy behaviors. This would be considered a reinforcement factor, and care must be taken when determining the difference between "healthy" and "unhealthy" for evaluating and monitoring public health programs, for example.

Assessments
Assessing individual and community health education needs provides the foundation for program planning and determines what health problems may exist in certain groups. It requires identifying community resources available to address the problem and encourages individuals to assume responsibility for and ownership of their health problems.

Assets Assessment
Planning health education strategies, interventions, and programs involves developing goals and objectives that are specific, measureable, and effective. Implementation is based on a thorough understanding of the priority population using a wide range of educational methods and techniques. Depending on the setting, used tests, surveys, observations, and tracking data, health educators use research to improve their program and practice, which involves facilitating cooperation among personnel and skills required to access resources and establish effective, consultative relationships. It may also involve translating scientific terminology and language into user-friendly information to address diverse groups or settings.

Community Asset Maps
"Asset Mapping" is derived from an "asset-based" approach to community development. It refers to a range of approaches that work from the principle that a community can be built only by focusing on the strengths and capacities of the citizens

and associations who call a neighborhood, community, or county 'home.' There are three areas to consider:

- Gifts, skills, and capacities of the individuals living in the community
- Citizen associations where local people gather to pursue common goals
- Institutions in the community such as hospitals, government offices, and education and human service agencies.

Needs Assessment

In needs assessments, health educators gather and analyze information to determine which health education program goals and strategies are appropriate for a specified target population. Individual needs may be basic, but essential for learning, growth, and development (e.g. food, water, shelter, warmth). They may, however, be more complex (e.g. sense of safety, security, emotional support, self-efficacy) and affected by multiple family, school, and community factors (e. g. family structure, available community resources, contribution opportunities).

Basic individual needs and/or complex family, school, and community needs indicate gaps between "what currently exists" and "what is optimal." Needs assessment is the systematic, planned collection of information about individuals' health-related knowledge, attitudes, beliefs, perceptions, motivations, skills, and behaviors, as well as environmental factors that may impact health. Health educators can conduct further comprehensive needs assessments examining existing health-related programs and resources in the surrounding community. Needs assessment is critical for designing relevant, appropriate, and culturally sensitive health education programs. Logically assessing needs precedes planning and implementing program goals and strategies.

The primary purpose of the curriculum is to promote, motivate, and assist individuals and groups in maintaining and improving their health, preventing disease, and minimizing risky health-related behaviors. It allows individuals and groups to develop and demonstrate health knowledge, skills, and practices. It can support health instruction integration into physical education, family and consumer science, guide program development, and other areas.

Physical Activity: Modeling and Encouraging the Achievement of Lifelong Physical Fitness

Quality physical education should promote, through a variety of planned physical activities, each student's optimum physical, mental, emotional, and social development and should offer activities and sports that students enjoy and can pursue throughout their lives. Qualified, trained instructors teach physical education. The school and community can promote the achievement and maintenance of a health-enhancing physical fitness level through an environment that supports physical activity opportunities.

Health Services: Enhancing School Health Services

Health services include services to appraise, protect, and promote health. These services are designed to ensure access or referral to primary healthcare services; prevent and control communicable disease and other health problems; provide emergency care for illness or injury; and promote and provide education and counseling opportunities to promote and maintain individual, family, and community health. Qualified professionals, such as physicians, school nurses, nurse practitioners, and other allied health personnel, provide these services.

Nutrition and Food Service: Encouraging Healthful Nutrition

Nutrition services include access to a variety of nutritious and appealing meals that accommodate student health and nutritional needs and reflect U.S. Dietary Guidelines. These services are designed to include culturally and medically appropriate foods that promote growth and development, pleasurable eating, and long-term health. Nutrition education is an integral part of the school nutrition program. Qualified child nutrition professionals provide these services.

Guidance and Counseling: Supporting Social and Emotional Well-being

School counseling, psychological, and mental health services work to improve students' mental, emotional, and social health. These services include education, individual and group assessments, interventions, and referrals. Professionals, such as certified school counselors, student assistance professionals, home-school coordinators, psychologists, and social workers, provide these services.

School Environment: Creating Positive Learning Environments

A healthy school environment includes safe and aesthetically pleasing equipment, buildings, and grounds; a culture that promotes an equitable, safe, and healthy climate for students; and policies, procedures, and conditions that support the well-being of students and staff. To learn and teach most effectively, students and staff must engage in settings where they feel safe, supported, and comfortable.

Steps for Planning the Needs Assessment Process

Step 1: Identify a Community Group

Identify community members to serve on a Community Group. Over the course of two meetings, group members will review data and information to identify and prioritize community health needs. When compiling the list of community members to serve on the Community Group, include 15 to 20 individuals who are viewed as community leaders representing the broad interests of the community across varying sectors (e.g. education, health, business, agriculture, faith). The group must include person(s) with special knowledge of or expertise in public health, as well as leaders, representatives, or members of medically underserved, low-income, and minority populations and populations with chronic disease. Some group members also may be asked to participate in one-on-one interviews.

Step 2: Collect and Review Data

While organizing and planning the Community Group, begin compiling secondary data to share with the Community Group to help inform its analysis and decisions. Sources for secondary data may include the U.S. Census Bureau, County Health

Rankings, and individual state departments of health. Typical secondary data related to a hospital's service area includes demographic information (such as population trends, age, poverty rates, educational attainment), the prevalence of health conditions and diseases, levels of insurance and other factors affecting access to care, clinical care measures, environmental factors, causes of death, rates of preventive measures, and information about children's health. Share basic demographic data about the hospital's service area at Meeting One of the Community Group; save the more detailed information for Meeting Two when the Community Group is reviewing survey results and making decisions about area health needs and priorities. For Meeting One, compile hospital information about how its service area was defined, its services and community benefits, and its economic impact.

Step 3: Convene the Community Group for Meeting One
On the agenda for Meeting One of the Community Group:
1. Introductions
2. Overview of the process
3. Define the hospital's service area
4. Explain the hospital's services, facilities, and community benefits
5. Share demographic data
6. Conduct focus group session further exploring the survey topics using a neutral facilitator (Explain the process for survey distribution to additional community members and discuss next steps: next meeting, additional survey distribution, etc.)

Step 4: Administer Survey to Community Members and Healthcare Professionals:
Develop two versions of a health needs assessment survey – one version for community members and one version for healthcare professionals. Distribute the surveys as widely as possible to area residents and healthcare professionals, taking care to make them available to different demographic groups, including lower-income residents, medically underserved residents, minority residents, and residents with chronic health conditions. Surveys may be distributed by electronic copy, by hard copy, or both. In this process, surveys are intended to be an additional tool for collecting qualitative information about community perceptions, not a method of collecting statistically valid data.

Step 5: Collect and Analyze Survey Data:
Hard-copy surveys should be returned via mail to ensure anonymity and confidentiality. Compile the data and prepare a report of the results. In the report, include the secondary data about health conditions and indicators gathered in Step 2. During this time, consider having a neutral party conduct a number of key informant interviews and include those findings in the report.

Step 6: Convene the Community Group for Meeting Two:
At Meeting Two, the Community Group will review survey results, findings of the focus group session in Meeting One and key informant interviews, and secondary data about health conditions and indicators. Based on this aggregated information, the

Community Group should prepare a list of community health needs and then prioritize those needs.

A typical agenda for Meeting Two of the Community Group is:
1. Review Meeting One
2. Present secondary data about health conditions and indicators
3. Present results of consumer survey and health professionals survey
4. Present findings of key interviews and focus group session from Meeting One
5. Develop list of community health needs
6. Prioritize identified health needs
7. Final comments

Step 7: Draft Community Health Needs Assessment Report:
Based on the decisions and recommendations of the Community Group, draft a Community Health Needs Assessment report that includes strategies for implementation. To ensure the appropriate information is collected, seek input from all required sources and document the methods as you progress.

Step 8: Draft Strategic Implementation:
After completing the needs assessment report, adopt and draft an implementation strategy that describes how the facility plans to meet the prioritized needs identified in the assessment.

Steps for Conducting a Needs Assessment
The first step in conducting a needs assessment is to identify credible sources of data. Interactive, web-based data query systems provide information and are used to identify health conditions and behaviors affecting the community and state. Credible sources of data include community data profiles that provide information relevant to health conditions, preventive screening, and health behaviors of interest. Conducting a needs assessment requires reviewing and analyzing the data and searching for disparities among demographic indicators like age, gender, race, income, education, and healthcare coverage.

A needs assessment may require local data to be collected to fill in gaps in the data sources. It might include environmental, safety, and policy factors in the community that are critically impact individual health. After gathering and analyzing data for the needs assessment, the next step is to prioritize the information and set goals.

Service Need Versus Service Demand
The healthcare system can be viewed as an interaction between trained personnel, equipment, and services (supply) and individuals, groups, and communities (demand). Interaction between the supply and demand groups can improve the users' health needs. People need information, affirmation, and support to articulate and exercise their rights when demanding these needed services.

5 Models for Conducting a Needs Assessment

Epidemiological Model involves an epidemiological diagnosis where you identify the health or other issues that most influence the outcome the community seeks. In this diagnosis, you create the objectives for your intervention.

Public Health Model involves a community needs assessment that builds interest and promotes working together to create an informed community and identify health issues and concerns through focus groups and surveys.

Social Model is used to evaluate assessments against a social model of disability to determine how effectively a project has met its objectives/goals. It can identify project barriers and help determine whether to continue the program or disseminate the findings.

Asset Model determines how to promote community health by assessing where the community stands. It allows community members to identify support and mobilize existing community resources to create a shared vision of change, and it encourages greater creativity when community members address problems and issues.

Rapid Model engages with initial community sectors in a process to grow into comprehensive assessments while providing additional opportunity to immediately address community health issues. It establishes partners in the community and a framework for health assessments. Information gathered will be aligned with the results of the community assessments, guidelines, and requests.

Health Impact Assessment (HIA) is defined as a combination of procedures, methods, and tools by which a policy, program, or project may be judged according to its potential effects on the health of a population and the distribution of those effects within that population. Assessment results are used in the planning process and identify desired outcomes through assessing the resources available to achieve goals and objectives. A planning model with measureable, attainable, and realistic goals should be selected. Identify and use strategies and interventions that ensure consistency within those objectives.

A **Data Analysis Plan** helps you understand the demographic, education, and socioeconomic indicators when identifying health needs and planning health programs. There are different types of analyses programs to consider:

A **meta-analysis** refers to methods that focus on contrasting and combining results from different studies to hopefully identify patterns among study results, sources of disagreement among those results, and other interesting relationships that may be revealed in multiple studies. In its simplest form, it is the identification of a common measure of size or weighted average that may be related to sample sizes within individual studies. The general aim of a meta-analysis is to more powerfully estimate the true effect of size as opposed to a less precise effect from a single study with a given set of conditions and assumptions. A meta-analysis is an important part of a systematic review procedure and may be conducted on several clinical trials of a medical treatment to understand how well it works. Meta-analysis combines evidence and forms part of a framework that relies on precision planning to guide data analysis.

Pooled data analysis is often used to provide an overall summary of subgroup data or data from a number of related studies. In simple pooling, data is combined without being weighted. Therefore, the analysis is performed as if the data was extracted from a single sample. This kind of analysis ignores characteristics of the pooled subgroups and individual studies and can yield false or counterintuitive results. In meta-analysis, data from subgroups and individual studies is first weighted and then combined, thereby avoiding some of the problems of simple pooling.

Data Collection Methods

Delphi Panels Process
The **Delphi method** is a structured communication technique, originally developed as a systematic, interactive forecasting method that relies on a panel of experts. The experts answer questionnaires in two or more rounds. After each round, a facilitator provides an anonymous summary of the experts' forecasts and explanations of their judgments. Thus, experts are encouraged to revise their earlier answers after reviewing other panel members' replies. It is believed that during this process, the range of answers will decrease, and the group will converge towards the "correct" answer. Finally, the process is stopped after a pre-defined stop criterion (e.g. number of rounds, achievement of consensus, stability of results), and the median scores of the final rounds determine the results.

Delphi is based on the principle that forecasts (or decisions) from a structured group of individuals are more accurate than those from unstructured groups. The technique can also be adapted for face-to-face meetings and is then called mini-Delphi or Estimate-Talk-Estimate (ETE). Delphi has been widely used for business forecasting and has certain advantages over other structured forecasting approaches such as predicting markets.

Nominal Group Process
The Nominal Group Technique (NGT) is an evaluative methodology that allows the generation of ideas and thoughts from group participants through the posing of a single question, while maintaining anonymity throughout. The process requires direct involvement from all participants, ensuring a democratic experience for all. It has the capacity to generate abundant data from only one session with participants, which highlights the cost-effectiveness of the approach.

Observation

Observation is a primary method of collecting data by human, mechanical, electrical, or electronic means with direct or indirect contact and involves careful looking and listening. We all watch other people sometimes, but we do not usually watch them to discover particular information about their behavior. Observation is the main source of information in field research, a process where a researcher observes conditions in their natural state.

There are many types of observation: direct or indirect, participant or non-participant, obtrusive or non-obtrusive, and structured or non-structured. Observation is important because natural behavior is observed instead of what people say they did or felt. For example, people value health, but they eat food they know is fatty. Observation is useful when the subject cannot provide information or can only provide inaccurate information, such as when people are addicted to drugs. However, when observing, the researcher does not receive insight into people's thoughts.

Probability
Probability is a realization, or observed value, of a random value that is actually observed or that is what actually happened in a given situation. The random variable should be considered as the process of how the observation comes about. Statistical quantities computed from realizations without deploying a statistical model are often called empirical or regarded as having empirical probability.

Non-probability
A non-probability sample is not based on random selection methods. The purpose of sampling is to obtain an accurate representation of the targeted population so to draw accurate conclusions. The samples are large and randomly drawn; every member of the population has a known, nonzero probability of being included in the sample. In simple random samples, every member would have an equal probability of being chosen, but there are also other variants. Often, random sampling is not possible or is too expensive. It requires a complete list of the population or some other way of guaranteeing that every member is considered, and selected units cannot be replaced if they are unavailable or refuse to participate.

Quota
Quota polling, a type of one-on-one sampling, is when a one-on-one interview is conducted by phone or in-person using a questionnaire. Today, this polling can be completed electronically for standardization, effectiveness, and instant results.

Convenience
Information collected from school programs can yield valuable information, which is conveniently taken from samplings or screenings for complete data.

Stratified Samples
Stratified samples are taken from a population divided into subgroups (strata). The groups are then sampled individually. Sample results may be evaluated individually or combined to estimate the characteristics of the total sample population. A more representative sample can be taken from a relatively homogenous population, which means fewer items must be studied when several strata are examined separately than

when the entire population is evaluated. Stratification improves the sampling process as various audit procedures can be applied to each stratum, depending on the situation. Stratification should be used when the characteristic under examination varies materially within portions of a population.

Inferential Statistics

Inferential statistics help you select tests, based on characteristics of the data collected, to interpret the results. Numerous kinds of statistical analysis can be performed in health information management. Using inferential statistics in health information management involves establishing an ordinal scale to evaluate coding accuracy to evaluate coders, for example, based on a scale of 1 to 4.

- Score 1 means the correct code was assigned for the principal diagnosis and only minor coding errors among secondary diagnoses.
- Score 2 means the correct code was assigned for the principal diagnosis, but there are omissions or major errors among secondary diagnoses.
- Score 3 means a minor coding error in the principal diagnosis and only minor errors in secondary diagnoses.
- Score 4 means a minor coding error in the principal diagnosis and major errors or omissions in secondary diagnoses.

Surveys

The purpose of health surveys is to disseminate pertinent information regarding the burden of disease and risk factor trends. Over the last several decades, health research has influenced mortality rates, advocating healthier lifestyles and engaging people in disease preventative activities. The effect that data quality has on these aspects depends on many factors. Ensuring reliability, accuracy of data tools, representative samples, and the validity of participant responses are the challenges faced when conducting health surveys.

Whether verbal or written, surveys are a method to understand public opinion and perceptions. In the wider realm of sociology, politics, economics, and behavioral psychology, and across industries, statistical research is used to uncover the underlying "truth." When conducting a research study, the design of data tools is as important as selecting the right methodological approaches. Appropriate attention should be given to properly developing the instruments used to collect data. Why? It is essential to avoid creating gaps between the theoretical postulates of research and the language used to find facts.

Design

When developing health survey questions, it is important to first determine the direction of your research. Take time to plan your survey questions so you can eliminate discrepancies in research results and generate focused, specified data. It is also important to use valid and reliable questions. Survey questions about health or health-related topics involve the following steps:

1. Decide how to measure the concepts

2. Relate the concepts to the survey design and objectives
3. Match the scale for the chosen measures to the analysis plan
4. Evaluate the reliability of the measures
5. Evaluate the validity of the measures
6. Choose the most appropriate method of data collection
7. Tailor the measures to the study sample
8. Determine the best way to ask the actual questions
   Step 8 involves three categories that will assist in focusing and creating the right type of questions to ask:
   - Problem/health issue
   - Target audience
   - Behavior specifically desired

Collect Data

Writing accurate questions is vital to collecting accurate data. Non-sampling errors can occur when writing questions by inadvertently leading respondents to provide a specific response. It is crucial to determine what needs to be studied and to know the concepts behind the questions being asked. For example, consider the phrase "the satisfaction with the work of the present management" versus "the amount of hours people work normally". The first question attempts to capture a feeling about the management, while the second is more factual information about work.

Plan Data Analysis

Before many research activities, pretesting or piloting questions in focus groups can prove to be beneficial in creating the right questions for specific issues. By identifying factors within the responses, it will help develop consistent data and will remove redundant questions. This ensures that respondents interpret the meaning of the questions as the researcher intended, which permits reliability testing and eliminates existing discrepancies and biases before field use.

Additionally, the context effect can influence survey responses since it can impact how respondents perceive and answer the questions. To make respondents comfortable, questions should be asked in an order of increasing sensitivity.

Drawing the Sample

At times, a researcher can get too involved with his/her study and blur the lines of the mandatory procedures. Especially when working with vulnerable populations or those with low levels of education, investigators may tend to impose their own beliefs, attitudes, and perceptions on respondents, thereby influencing questions and behavior. However, questions can be framed in a way that ensures respondents are providing responses reflective of their personal beliefs.

For example, an original survey question might be: "Are you aware that people are testing a vaccine against hook worm? **Concerns about this survey question:** Firstly, this type of information should be included in the informed consent given to every participant before voluntarily participating in the study. Secondly, including the correct response in the question leads a higher proportion of respondents to agree with it. The question does not assess whether the respondent was actually aware that researchers were testing a vaccine against hookworm. A **re-phrased survey question would ask:** "Do you know what is being tested?" If the respondent replies "yes," the next question should ask: "What is being tested?"

Construct Survey
Personalization may improve response rates to surveys, but it may also result in a higher number of socially desirable responses. An option for preventing bias questions may result in questions that provide a response of "no opinion." However, beware that this option can also profoundly affect data quality. Including this type of answer choice doesn't increase data quality and can often eliminate the opportunity to capture significant information or opinions.

Sources of potential bias in non-response questions mainly occur when asking about health behaviors (i.e. physical activity, smoking, drug and alcohol use, wearing condoms, wearing helmets or seatbelts, use of insecticide-treated bed nets, etc.), social status (primarily income), witnessing violent acts, and gender or age differences (male versus female responders). Large budgets and more funding do not always create a higher-quality survey. Good survey design requires and uses the same fundamental principles regardless of the survey size.

Remember, cultural values provide important insights, and these nuances are also important to research results. Therefore, reducing or controlling socially desirable biases may be inappropriate in some instances. Refer to similar studies for conceptual frameworks to help guide the development and selection of survey material. By reviewing similar articles and questionnaires, a relevant summary of research methods and results can be provided, but remember that published research studies in peer-reviewed journals do not necessarily use quality survey design, and it is therefore important to carefully consider the validity of each question in a research study.

Appropriate interview techniques have an impact on the quality of results, especially when working cross-culturally and in different languages. Overall, valid data can help develop policy and provide the opportunity to design and implement culturally appropriate interventions.

Pretest Survey
The efficacy of research that relies on incredible, self-reported data attempts to use a more objective approach to obtain accurate measurements. Strategies to reduce study bias in a pretest survey include:
- Comparing subjective and objective data and highlighting deficiencies in the collected subjective data
- Conducting anonymous self-administered questionnaires
- Providing participants with methods that ensure privacy and confidentiality.

Revise Survey

Health surveys have been and will continue to be important sources of information for healthcare policymakers, public health professionals, private providers, insurers, and healthcare consumers concerned with planning, implementing, and evaluating health-related programs and policies. The design and conduct of future health surveys will be shaped by changes in the diversity, complexity, and sensitivity of the topics addressed in current studies; the innovative techniques and technologies being developed for administering them; and the new or intensified ethical dilemmas resulting from these changes. By creating and conducting health surveys firmly based on quality techniques, researchers of today can help shape the outcomes of tomorrow.

Seven Steps of Survey Analysis

Qualitative research methods are used primarily by social scientists to investigate human behavior. The advantages of qualitative research are that it provides in-depth information and is a good investigative tool for obscure subjects. Although interviews, focus groups, and reviews are the primary modes of investigation for qualitative research, surveys may also be used. While quantitative research uses surveys to create statistics, qualitative surveys will create more in-depth knowledge that will be analyzed using a more deductive process.

Step 1 - Perform Data Reduction:
Even with survey results, qualitative research often amasses a large amount of raw data, which must be filtered and organized. This process involves selecting, focusing, simplifying, and transforming the data. Survey data, as opposed to transcripts from interviews or processing groups, is already organized to some extent. This process should include highlighting important parts of the data, and physically sorting, coding, or highlighting the data into initial categories.

Step 2 - Group Data into Meaningful Patterns and Themes:
Consider these patterns in terms of the larger questions of your study and whether the data supports or refutes these questions. If not, why not? Based on what you see in the data, you may process it using content analysis, which includes coding the data for certain words or content, identifying patterns, and interpreting meaning. Or it may require a more thematic analysis, which groups data into themes in an effort to answer research questions.

Step 3 - Create a Data Display:
Data display is the process of transforming data into a visual format. You may choose to create a chart, matrix, diagram, graph, or table. This display should help arrange the data in new ways and help analyze and identify emerging patterns and meanings in the content.

Step 4 - Draw Conclusions about the Data:
This step involves backtracking, interpreting the data, and considering its meanings and implications according to your original research questions.

<u>Step 5 - Verify Your Analysis</u>:
Verification involves revisiting the data to confirm the conclusions you've made. This step may involve reviewing the data multiple time

<u>Step 6 - Have Another Person or Researcher Help with the Process</u>:
This assistance may be particularly helpful in the verification process.

<u>Step 7 - Use Computer Software to Assist in Qualitative Data Analysis</u>:
These programs may be helpful in organizing data; however, they do not produce the themes and meanings that human analysis provides. They are also expensive and require time and resources to use them.

Types of Surveys

A survey is a way of collecting information that you hope represents the views of the entire targeted community or group. Surveys are usually written, although sometimes, the surveyor reads the questions aloud and writes down the answers for another person. They can be distributed by mail, fax, e-mail, or a web page, or the questions can be asked over the phone or in person.

Surveys collect information in as uniformly a manner as possible, asking each respondent the same questions in the same way to ensure answers are most influenced by the respondents' experiences, not how the interviewer words the questions. Here are some different types of surveys:

Mail Surveys
1. *Case study surveys* collect information from a part of a group or community without sampling them for overall representation of the larger population. You may need to conduct several of these surveys before you understand how the larger community might respond. Case study surveys only provide specific information about the community studied.

2. *Sampled surveys* are the type that asks questions to a sample portion of a group. If done correctly, the sample results will reflect the results you would have received by surveying the entire group. For example, if you wanted to know what percentage of people in your county uses an adult literacy program, getting 10,000 people to complete a survey would be a huge task. Instead, you decide to survey a sample of 500 people to discover what they think. For the sample to accurately represent the larger group, it must be chosen carefully.

3. *Census surveys* are when you distribute your survey questionnaire to every member of a population. This method will produce the most accurate information about the group, but it may not be very practical for large groups. A census is best done with smaller groups -- all of the clients of a particular agency, for example, as opposed to all of the residents of a city.

Telephone Surveys

Telephone surveys of public health research have increased. Firstly, telephone interviews are highly recommended for follow-up interviews in panel surveys that use an initial face-to-face interview. Secondly, telephone surveys are recommended as a viable alternative to costly face-to-face surveys in cross-sectional studies of the general population. Thirdly, when the survey focuses on subgroups of the population with low telephone coverage and high rates of non-response (e.g. low income and low education respondents), telephone interviews should be used more cautiously. In these situations, a dual-sampling frame approach (using a combination of face-to-face and telephone interviewing) may be considered. Finally, computer-assisted telephone interviewing (CATI) represents one of the most important and innovative technological advances in health survey research in recent years. The advantages of CATI in improving survey management are noteworthy, and this process is ideally suited for moderate- to large-sample surveys. CATI also provides an attractive (and largely untapped) resource for testing and refining other method protocols of survey research.

In-Person Survey

Focus Groups	Surveys
Require larger time commitment from participants	Require relatively shorter time commitment from participants
Require advance planning to invite guests, reserve space, develop questions, etc.	Require advance planning to develop questions, distribute surveys, and process answers
Acquire information from a relatively small group of representative stakeholders	Acquire information from an entire group (depending on size) or a large sample; can be given to unlimited numbers of people
Use a trained facilitator	Do not require a trained facilitator
Allow participants to build on each other's ideas	Participants do not have the ability to build on each other's ideas
Occurs at a fixed time and in a set manner	Can be administered in a variety of ways (verbal or written, in person, or via phone or mail) and over a period of time
Participants provide information, but may also become more informed in the process.	Participants can provide information, but it is not always easy to provide them with information
Public environments can intimidate some participants	Written surveys may present problems for lower-level readers
Feedback is immediate	Getting surveys returned may be a problem
Allow participants to ask for clarification	Survey questions may be misinterpreted

Allow participants to elaborate or explain their answers	Survey questions can be open-ended or multiple choice; multiple choice questions are easier to summarize, but the data may not be as rich

Primary, Secondary, and Tertiary Data and Sources

Various professional fields treat the distinction between primary and secondary sources in differing fashions. Some fields and references also further distinguish between secondary and tertiary sources. Primary, secondary, and tertiary sources are defined below.

Primary sources are close to the source or origin of a particular topic or event. An eyewitness account of a traffic accident is an example of a primary source. Other examples include archeological artifacts; photographs; videos; historical documents, such as diaries, census results, maps, transcripts of surveillance, public hearings, trials, and interviews; un-tabulated results of surveys or questionnaires; the original written or recorded notes of laboratory and field research, experiments or observations unpublished in a peer-reviewed source; original philosophical works, religious scripture, administrative documents, patents, and artistic and fictional works, such as poems, scripts, screenplays, novels, motion pictures, videos, and television programs.

Secondary sources are at least one step removed from an event or body of primary-source material and may include an interpretation, analysis, or synthetic claims about the subject. Secondary sources may use primary sources and other secondary sources to create a general overview or to make analytic or synthetic claims.

Tertiary sources are publications, such as encyclopedias or other compendia that summarize secondary and primary sources. For example, *Wikipedia* is a tertiary source. Many introductory textbooks may also be considered tertiary because they summarize multiple primary and secondary sources.

Quantitative versus Qualitative Data

The methods and data produced are grouped into 2 categories – quantitative and qualitative. Quantitative methods produce hard numbers, while qualitative methods provide more descriptive data using words. The chosen methods are determined by the purpose of your evaluation and the resources used to design and conduct it. Using both quantitative and qualitative data is commonly referred to as a "mixed method" and produces a more comprehensive understanding of a project's goals and achievements.

Quantitative Techniques include:
- Surveys
- Questionnaires
- Pre and post-tests
- Existing databases
- Statistical analysis

Qualitative Techniques include:
- Observations
- Interviews
- Focus groups
- Non-statistical methods

Research Methods

Research Methods covers the entire research process including: formulating research questions, sampling (probability and non-probability), measurement (surveys, scaling, qualitative, and unobtrusive), research design (experimental and quasi-experimental), data analysis, and research writing. It also addresses research validity, measurement reliability, and ethics.

Key Informant Interviews

Key informants' commitment to health equity is clearly reflected in their definitions of healthcare challenges and needed actions. There are insufficiencies, inequities, and limitations of the current healthcare system including environmental factors and individual approaches to achieving the highest health level for all people. Communities identified by respondents as the most affected by health disparities include Latinos, Asians (specifically Vietnamese, Laotian, and Cambodian), and racial minorities. Among these groups, chronic disease and obesity are described as the most common health issues.

Having sufficient services to meet residents' needs helps equalize health conditions. Health equity is further realized when all community members can go anywhere for care. This situation requires a system-wide capacity for providing culturally appropriate services in a client's primary language. It also requires adequate care for residents facing multiple health challenges or needing specialized care. The entire community is better served when providers work holistically in a client-centered environment. By linking healthcare systems, we are better able to connect with people throughout their healthcare journey. This connection enhances individual capacity to make healthful choices, access appropriate care, and receive the support they need to prevent disease progression and hospital visits.

Errors

Research versus Systematic

Random errors can be evaluated through statistical analysis and can be reduced by averaging a high number of observations. **Systematic errors** are difficult to detect and cannot be analyzed statistically because all data skewed in the same direction (either too high or too low). Spotting and correcting systematic errors requires focus.

Confounding Variables

In any experiment, many kinds of variables will affect results. The independent variable is the manipulation for the experiment, and the dependent variable is the measure from that experiment. Confounding variables affect the dependent variable, but are considered when designing the experiment. For example, if you want to know if Drug X causes drowsiness, the experimenter must carefully design the experiment to ensure the study subjects fall asleep because of the influence of Drug X and not because of other factors. Those other factors would be confounding variables.

Resource Inventory

Morbidity and Mortality Weekly Report (MMWR)

The goal of this report is to be (Centers For Disease Control) CDC's primary voice for scientific publication of timely, reliable, authoritative, accurate, objective, and useful science-based public health information and recommendations to those in need of the information.

The objective of MMWR is to describe current (timely, reliable, authoritative, accurate, objective, and useful science-based) public health information, provide recommendations based on that information, and describe how the recommendations will impact public health.

NCHS

National Center for Health Statistics (NCHS) showcases the capabilities and achievements of NCHS in the fields of health, health data, and health statistics. They hold conferences each year and include hands-on workshops, educational sessions, and exhibits.

Centers for Disease Control (CDC)

Today's state-of-the-art health education curricula reflect growing research that emphasizes:
- Teaching essential, functional health information
- Shaping personal values and beliefs that support healthy behaviors
- Shaping group norms that value a healthy lifestyle
- Developing essential health skills necessary to adopt, practice, and maintain health-enhancing behaviors

U.S. Department of Health and Human Services

President Jimmy Carter created the U.S. Department of Health and Human Services in 1980 when the Department of Education was derived from the education component of the Department of Health, Education, and Welfare. The Department of Health and Human Services is led by the Secretary of Health and Human Services Staff Offices (e.g. general counsel; Assistant Secretaries for Health, for Legislation, for Planning and Evaluation, for Public Affairs, and for Management and Budget; and Director of the Office of Civil Rights), an independent inspector general, and twelve operating divisions:
1. Administration on Aging
2. Administration for Children and Families
3. Healthcare Financing Administration (Medicare and Medicaid)
4. Program Support Center

5. Agency for Healthcare Quality and Research
6. Agency for Toxic Substances and Disease Registry
7. Centers for Disease Control and Prevention (CDC)
8. Food and Drug Administration (FDA)
9. Health Resources and Services Administration
10. Indian Health Service
11. National Institutes of Health
12. Substance Abuse and Mental Health Services Administration

CSH

The CMS Coordinated School Health (CSH) Program uses the "whole child" approach to support teachers, parents, and communities to meet the physical, emotional, social, and educational needs of students. Together, we can help all students become healthy, educated, and productive adults. Benefits of CSH include:

- Reduced school absenteeism
- Improved student behavior
- Improved student performance
- Implemented policies and programs that support the inclusion of health education and awareness
- New levels of cooperation and collaboration among families, teachers, schools, health officials, and the community through school health advisory councils and school-based health teams

The eight components of the CSH Program that can be found in all CMS schools are:

1. Health Services:
   Provides prevention, education, emergency care, referrals, and management of health problems and is designed to minimize problems that interfere with learning.

2. Health Education:
   Provides classroom instruction that addresses physical, emotional, and social needs to improve student health and reduce risk behaviors.

3. Physical Education and Activity:
   Provides a planned, sequential Pre-K to 12 curriculum that teaches developmentally appropriate skills and promotes lifelong activity. A minimum of 30 minutes physical activity per day is required for grades K-8.

4. Nutrition Services:
   Integrates nutritious, affordable meals and nutrition education in an environment that promotes healthful eating.

5. Counseling, Psychological, and Social Services:
   Supports social and emotional well-being and helps schools respond to crises.

6. Healthy School Environment:
   Supports policies and facilities that create safe, secure, and healthy settings for positive learning experiences.

7. Human Resources and Services Administration (HRSA):
   HRSA supplies grants to organizations to improve and expand healthcare services for underserved people.

8. Social Security Administration (SSA)

Youth Risk Behavior Surveillance System (YRBSS)
The YRBSS monitors six types of health-risk behaviors that are considered the leading causes of death and disability among youth and adults including:
1. Behaviors that contribute to unintentional injuries and violence
2. Sexual behaviors that contribute to unintended pregnancy and sexually transmitted diseases including HIV infection
3. Alcohol and other drug use
4. Tobacco use
5. Unhealthful dietary behaviors
6. Inadequate physical activity

YRBSS also measures the prevalence of obesity and asthma among youth and young adults.

YRBSS includes a national, school-based survey conducted by the CDC and state, territorial, tribal, and local surveys conducted by state, territorial, and local education and health agencies.

Health and Psychosocial Instruments (HaPI) Database
Health and Psychosocial Instruments (HaPI) is a database that provides access to information on approximately 15,000 measurement instruments including questionnaires, interview schedules, checklists, coding schemes, and rating scales in the fields of health and psychosocial sciences. HaPI can be used to:
- Discover instruments
- Determine availability of reliable and valid evidence
- Track the history of an instrument over time
- Identify other instruments that have already developed in your field of study
- Locate ordering information for a known instrument

Database information is abstracted from hundreds of leading journals covering health sciences and psychosocial sciences. Additionally, instruments from industrial/organizational behavior and education are included.

The Health Insurance Portability and Accountability Act of 1996 (HIPAA)
The Office for Civil Rights enforces the HIPAA Privacy Rule, which protects individually identifiable health information. The HIPAA Security Rule sets national

security standards for electronically protected health information along with the Patient Safety Rule confidentiality provisions, which protect identifiable information used to analyze patient safety events and improve patient safety.

IRB

An **institutional review board (IRB)**, also known as an **independent ethics committee** or **ethical review board**, is a committee that has been formally designated to approve, monitor, and review human biomedical and medical research. They often conduct some form of risk/benefit analysis to determine whether or not to perform research. The number one priority of IRBs is to protect human subjects from physical or psychological harm.

In the U.S., the FDA and Department of Health and Human Services have empowered IRBs to approve, modify planned research prior to approval, or disapprove research. IRBs are responsible for critical 'scientific', 'ethical', and 'regulatory' oversight functions for human research.

Statistical Abstract of the United States

The *Statistical Abstract of the United States*, published since 1878, is the authoritative and comprehensive summary of statistics on the social, political, and economic organization of the U.S. The Abstract can be used as a convenient volume for statistical reference and as a guide to further informational sources in print and on the Web. Sources include the Census Bureau, Bureau of Labor Statistics, Bureau of Economic Analysis, and several other Federal agencies and private organizations.

Public Computerized Reference Databases

Health education specialists locate and obtain valid and reliable data about a specific population. Most health education specialists identify needs of the priority population by reviewing current literature. Literature databases are available in libraries (computer databases) and on the Internet. It is important that data refer to a population characteristically similar to the priority population.

BRFSS

The Behavioral Risk Factor Surveillance System (BRFSS) is the largest, continuous telephone health survey in the world. It enables the Centers for Disease Control and Prevention (CDC), state health departments, and other health agencies to monitor modifiable risk factors for chronic diseases and other leading causes of death. BRFSS data files are freely available in formats used by people trained to use statistical software to answer health research questions.

PubMed

PubMed comprises more than 22 million citations of biomedical literature from MEDLINE, life science journals, and online books. Citations may include links to full-text content from PubMed Central and publisher websites.

Education Resource Information Center (ERIC)
The list of journals includes titles indexed from 1966 to the present and indicates breaks in coverage (e.g. 1999-2001, 2004-current). The term "current" indicates that ERIC is actively indexing the journal. Record availability for an issue depends on publisher-provided content.

Journals currently indexed in ERIC are marked with an orange diamond. ERIC broadly defines "journal" as a regularly published periodical or serial publication with a stated aim and scope. ERIC lists, by series title, selected Monographic Series on the Non-Journal Source List.

Chapter 2: Plan Health Education

The purpose of planning is to ensure that the teaching is:
- Consistent with the domain of knowledge; level of the domain; individual or group preferences; learning styles; and cultural, ethnic, religious, and age-related needs
- Appropriate and specific to the identified learning needs
- Able to be evaluated in terms of effectiveness
- Modified according to any identified barriers to learning

The planning of health education must be complete, accurate, and collaboratively agreed to and participated in by the learner.

Planning consists of several components including:
- Developing learning objectives that are consistent with the domain of learning
- Deciding on a teaching strategy that is consistent with the domain of learning
- Planning content and learning activities that are consistent with the domain of learning and client needs
- Deciding upon and preparing for the use of learning resources, such as a medical model, a video tape, reading material, etc.
- Determining the length or duration of the teaching/learning session or episode

Priority Populations and Other Stakeholders in the Planning Process

Community Organization
Health educators play an important role in community advocacy and health education. Communities and populations are organized in a number of complex and diverse ways. For example, some communities are organized by ethnic and cultural patterns, while others are organized according to socioeconomic status; others are organized in terms of age. For example, some communities consist of young families with children, and senior citizens predominantly live in others.

Simply stated, populations consist of groups of people who share some characteristic that is discretely different from that of others outside of the population. Community can be defined as a group of people who interact with each other and have shared concerns and interests. Members of the community work collaboratively and collectively to address and resolve their common concerns and issues, including those relating to health and wellness.

An aggregate is a subpopulation or subgroup of a larger population. Aggregates share a common characteristic that links the people of the aggregate together. For example, an aggregate can consist of school age children who are linked by age or of a group of people who have the same disease or risk factor. For example, cigarette smokers are an aggregate with a common health-related risk factor.

The family unit is also a population within the larger community. Family is defined as a group of interconnected individuals who are connected with marriage, some other union, birth, cohabitation, or adoption. Members of the family unit interact with each other to perform family roles and functions and to collectively fulfill family responsibilities.

Priority Populations and Other Stakeholders
The purposes of planning are to prioritize needs and problems; to decide which needs can be met by the health educator; to develop a prioritized plan of action; and to decide upon long-term, intermediate, and short-term goals and behavioral objectives for educational activities.

Resources, whether they are material, time, and/or money, are limited. For this reason, priorities must be established. The first step is the prioritization of community health needs. Maslow's Hierarchy of Needs is often used as the framework for establishing priorities. This theory, or model, states that unless the lowest needs in this hierarchy are adequately satisfied, the higher needs cannot be met. The steps, or levels, of this hierarchy from the most basic and essential to the highest are the physical or biological needs, the need for safety and security, the need for love and belonging, the need for self-esteem and esteem by others, and the self-actualization needs. Health educators often focus on the lowest, most basic physical needs and the second priority, which is safety and security. For example, a health educator can plan and implement a nutritional education program for teens and a course on the need for bicycle helmets to prevent serious injuries among school age children.

Biological health includes not only freedom from disease, but also other characteristics, such as a healthful lifestyle, adequate housing, and sanitation. Psychological health consists of a high quality of life and mental health; social well-being can include such things as access to healthcare by all members of the population.

Additionally, some assessed needs are of immediate need, while others may be intermediate or long-term needs. Immediate, life-threatening needs are of the highest priority, and actual problems take priority over potential health-related problems.

Communicating the Need for Health Education to Priority Populations and Other Stakeholders
After educational needs are assessed and prioritized, these needs must be communicated to the affected groups, or priority population, and other stakeholders. A number of different mechanisms and forums can be used to communicate these needs. For example, the local school district can facilitate your communication with priority populations when the need for immunization education is identified; a senior center can communicate needs related to "sharing" prescribed medications with friends and family members; and a local civic group can assist with communicating the need for volunteers to drive disabled seniors to medical care, which would not be accessible without this assistance.

Collaboration with Priority Populations and Other Stakeholders and Eliciting Input

Unlike childhood learners, adult learners must be actively engaged and involved in all aspects of the teaching/learning process, including the planning phase, in collaboration with the health educator. Input must be elicited from the potential learners to ensure success.

The health educator typically forms a small group, representative of the priority population, to collaboratively plan the educational activity. Leading groups requires knowledge, skill, and abilities relating to group process, conflict and conflict resolution, and negotiation.

Some of the concepts relating to groups include the stages, or phases, of group process, including the:
- Forming, or orientation, stage
- Norming, or accommodation, stage
- Negotiation stage
- Operation and dissolution stage

Forming stage
The forming stage is the first stage of group development. Also referred to as the orientation stage, it is during this stage that members are selected, goals are established, and orientation to the group occurs.

Norming stage
The norming stage, also called the accommodation stage, focuses on decision-making, which can be done in a number of ways, including majority vote, consensus, etc.

Negotiation stage
This stage consists of task assignments and the assumption of roles, among other things.

Operation and dissolution stage
The operation stage involves the performance of roles and tasks to achieve group goals. The dissolution stage is the evaluation of the group's progress and the cessation of the group as it is.

Storming stage
The storming, or conflict, stage is included in some group process theories and is based on the fact that conflicts often occur in groups. Contrary to popular belief, conflicts can be resolved, and they are often productive rather than destructive.

Obtaining Commitments from Priority Populations and Other Stakeholders
Health promotion in the community aims to empower communities to prevent disease, to diagnose and treat disorders at their earliest stage with screening, and to alter risk patterns and behaviors. Populations will commit to these educational efforts when they

believe that the educational need exists and when they believe they can solve these health problems with education and behavioral changes.

Education, advocacy, empowerment, and behavior modification are components of health promotion. Potential solutions, or interventions, relating to identified problems may be at the primary, secondary, or tertiary level of prevention. Primary prevention aims to prevent the occurrence of health problems, disease, and dysfunction before it occurs. Secondary prevention involves the early identification and treatment of specific health problems. Tertiary prevention aims to return the client to the highest possible level of functioning following the correction of a health problem.

Developing Goals and Objectives

Identifying Desired Outcomes
Through the analysis of needs assessment data, an agenda can be set up for desired outcomes. The analysis is not always easy, as the results may not always appear in a straightforward manner. Identifying "what is" in a needs assessment does not always clearly show "what should be."

Desired outcomes, also referred to as learning goals, must be specific, measurable, behavioral, learner-centered, consistent with assessed need, and congruent with the domain of learning.

The three domains of learning, which are identified during the planning phase of the health education, include the following:
- Cognitive domain (also known as the thinking domain)
- Psychomotor domain (also known as the doing domain)
- Affective domain (also known as the feeling domain)

The cognitive domain is comprised of remembering or recalling previously learned material, comprehension, and application of knowledge. The cognitive domain of learning objectives includes the verbs *define*, *list*, *state*, *describe*, *summarize*, and *discuss*.

The psychomotor domain addresses the learner's need to do something. For example, the learner will watch a skill being done and then will practice it under the guidance of the health educator. The psychomotor domain includes the verbs *perform*, *use*, *manipulate*, and *demonstrate*.

The best way to write learning objectives is to begin the list of learning objectives with the statement, "At the conclusion of the teaching, the learner will be able to:" and then start the statement with a measurable verb that is consistent with the domain of learning and domain level. For example, "The learner will list all of the food groups," "The learner will be able to demonstrate relaxation techniques," and "The learner will perform CPR" are well-worded, specific, measurable, learner-centered learning objectives.

Determining Needed Resources

Human, material, and financial resources are needed for health education activities. Some of the possible resources that may be needed for various types of health education teaching can include instructors, assistants, set-up and clean-up crews, space for the learners, equipment, time (including preparation time, teaching time, and clean-up time), and money (including costs related to set-up, clean-up, necessary books or handouts, equipment, screens and technology for PowerPoint presentations, and medical equipment).

Designing Teaching Strategies and Interventions

Teaching strategies are determined according to the expected outcomes, the domain of learning, and the learning styles and preferences of the learners. Some people learn best by listening, some by watching, some by reading, and some by doing. Likewise, many learners prefer a videotape presentation over reading materials; others dislike watching television and viewing videotapes. Some like to read, while others do not. Many also benefit from, and enjoy, learning on the Internet; others are "computer-phobic." Some enjoy learning in small groups; others prefer privacy and one-to-one discussions.

Whenever possible, these individual learning styles and preferences should be accommodated for during the planning phase of the teaching/learning process. For example, if the assessment reveals that a patient or family member has a preference for a live one-to-one discussion about the impact of stress on blood glucose levels, these preferences must be accommodated.

Each domain has its own learning interventions and strategies. Strategies appropriate to the cognitive domain include peer group learning, lecture, discussion, online learning, computer-assisted learning, and independent reading. Some of the strategies for the psychomotor domain are live demonstration, videotaped demonstration, and step-by-step instructions.

Legal and Ethical Principles

Some of the ethical considerations for health educators include the presentation of current and scientifically sound principles and concepts, without any bias or coercion. All content must be valid and sound. Health educators must research the topic and develop content that is based on current medical literature. Additionally, all humans are unique, and they have the right to make autonomous decisions without any coercion. They are free to use, or not use, the information that is presented to them. Health educators must be supportive of client decisions regardless of whether or not the health educator thinks that these choices or decisions are the best for the client. Lastly, all educators must be ethically honest, fair, and respectful.

Some of the legal principles that impact health education include reasonable accommodation for those with a disability and non-discrimination. All learners are entitled to be taught in an environment that treats all learners the same, regardless of their age, race, religion, sexual orientation, or anything else. People with disabilities must also be accommodated. For example, wheelchair-bound and physically handicapped clients should not be confronted with physical barriers that prevent their participation in an educational activity. People with visual impairments should be provided large print reading materials and seating that can overcome this impairment. Those with a hearing impairment can benefit from a sign language interpreter, when feasible.

Cultural Competency

Ethnicity is often confused with culture, but is actually quite different. Ethnicity is defined as a group of racially similar people of a similar origin, whereas culture is defined as a group of people who have shared values, ideals, and beliefs, regardless of their race and ethnicity.

Communication patterns, vocabulary, and terminology are all things that must be considered in all teaching situations. There are differences between cultures in addition to language differences. The manner or way with which something is phrased can be understood very differently among different cultures. Therefore, it is vital that when planning a teaching session, the learner's cultural comprehension and level of understanding are thoroughly incorporated into the teaching process.

All cultures have a unique vocabulary, slang, and/or terminology. For example, if you are teaching a health education class at a predominantly Hispanic high school, it is important to use terms and terminology that are familiar to adolescents and the Hispanic culture. Generally speaking, medical terminology, such as "NPO," and complex medical descriptions should not be used. Health educators must be culturally competent about specific cultures and their norms and gestures and must modify their terminology and behavior according to what is acceptable and understandable to the learner.

Pilot Testing Strategies and Interventions and Using Findings to Refine and Improve the Educational Plan
It is suggested that, when possible, all educational activities be pilot tested with a small group before being implemented in a larger, formal group. Pilot testing allows the health educator to critically evaluate the educational session and make necessary changes to improve it.

There are two types of evaluation that should be done during pilot testing. They are referred to as formative and summative evaluation. Formative evaluation is the continuous assessment of the effectiveness of the teaching while the teaching is actually being conducted. This allows the teacher to modify the plan during the actual teaching session, as indicated. Summative evaluation occurs at the end of the learning activity and allows the health educator to determine whether or not the education has achieved the established learning objectives for the individual or group.

At times, the pilot or trial educational activity may need only slight revisions and improvements, but at other times, more extensive changes may be needed.

The Scope and Sequence for the Health Education

Even the most experienced health educators have problems with accurately planning the duration and scope of a teaching session. The scope of the teaching depends on what the individual or group knows or can do before the teaching and what you want the person to know or do after the teaching session, as stated in the learning objectives. For example, if you are teaching a group of mothers about immunizations and you have assessed that this population is not knowledgeable about the routine immunization schedule, the importance of immunization, or about where to get these immunizations, the scope of this activity will include at least these three content areas (immunization schedule, importance of immunizations, and where the mothers can get their baby immunized).

Some of the factors that can impact the amount of time needed to effectively facilitate learning include:
- Attention span: Children, the cognitively impaired, and those with serious illness and pain have a short attention span. Teaching/learning sessions for these patients and family members should be brief and modified, as based on the individual's need.

- Time: Heterogeneous (mixed groups with varying levels of knowledge) and large groups tend to require more time for a teaching session than do homogeneous (similar group members in terms of knowledge) and small groups.

The health educator must allow enough time for questions (cognitive domain) and return demonstration (psychomotor domain).

The sequencing of the educational activity should be planned so the learners can move from what is known and familiar to them to the unknown and unfamiliar (the learning objective). Adults have a wealth of knowledge and experience to draw upon. How long will it take to move learners from their previously held cognitive knowledge about immunizations to the point that the learners understand the importance of immunizations and initiate a behavioral change that involves having their children vaccinated?

Sequencing content also moves from the simple to the complex and from the non-threatening to the threatening. For example, how long will it take to move learners from knowledge about the need for blood glucose monitoring to actually performing a finger stick on themselves without fear or anxiety?

Selecting Resources

It is important to know that all learners are not at the same educational level. Some learners have advanced college degrees, and others may have only completed high school or hold only a GED. Some clients are literate and able to read, and others are not. Some may also have a language barrier that impedes the reading and comprehension of English. Some may be health literate, whereas others are not. Health-literate clients are able to understand information and use it to make appropriate healthcare decisions. Almost 50% of patients are not health literate. Health educators must modify their communication and teaching to accommodate this weakness and to ensure comprehension among these learners.

In addition to learning styles and personal preferences, materials must also be carefully selected.

Integrating Health Education into Other Programs

Health education can often times be integrated into other programs and in a wide variety of other forums, in addition to the traditional healthcare setting. Schools, state departments of health, corporations, civic groups, religious and church groups, and community health fairs are a few examples. The possibilities are limited only by our creativity.

Health education can become part of the larger curriculum for children in elementary schools, high schools, and colleges and universities. Corporations and industries, such as manufacturing for example, have a need for wellness education. Corporations are beginning to understand that wellness programs increase employee productivity and decrease costs associated with health insurance and absenteeism. Civic and religious groups are also excellent forums for educational activities. Many of these groups share common wellness and health-related educational needs that can be fulfilled by the health educator. For example, members of these groups may need education relating to the Affordable Care Act. Lastly, health fairs offer health educators a wide variety of educational opportunities to present educational activities to members of the local community.

Addressing Factors that Affect Implementation

Health educators also identify and analyze factors that foster or hinder implementation. Once these barriers are identified, they must be addressed and eliminated. Barriers to learning include physical, cognitive, sensory, and psychological barriers.

There are a number of physical barriers that can prevent the teaching/learning process. For example, the learner may be unable to physically get to his/her class due to a disability or the lack of transportation. It is then necessary to analyze this problem and determine an appropriate solution.

Cognitive and comprehension barriers can be accommodated with slow speech, the use of simple and understandable explanation, time for clarification and re-clarification, repetition, and the use of pictures and diagrams.

Sensory barriers can be eliminated with, for example, the use of Braille reading materials for the blind, speaking loudly for the auditory impaired, and the use of large print materials for the visually impaired.

Emotional and psychological barriers, such as fear and anxiety, can be overcome when the health educator establishes trust; maintains an open, trusting environment; positively rewards learning with praise; and attempts to alleviate any anxiety. Mild anxiety promotes learning; severe anxiety prohibits learning.

An Environment that is Conducive to Learning

When developing an environment that is conducive to learning, several physical and non-physical environmental factors must be considered. The age of the learners, the content of the learning, the number of learners in the group, the size of the room where the teaching will occur, etc. are all factors that must be considered during the planning process.

An ideal environment is one that is environmentally comfortable. The temperature of the room should be set at a level that is not too warm, where a student or teacher may perspire, and not too cool, where they may feel chilled. The room should be well lit to allow students to view things, such as white boards, chalkboards, or any other visual displays. There also should be a mechanism to dim the lights for things, such as PowerPoint presentations, videos, etc.

Seating is another aspect that should be considered. For example, a group of comfortable chairs arranged in a circle can be appropriate for small groups when note taking is not necessary. Chairs with a small desk attached or a round table surrounded by comfortable chairs can be used when note taking and small group work are part of the educational activity.

Non-environmental factors that impact learning include the interpersonal relationship of the healthcare educator and the learners. All learning must be conducted in an environment that is open; accepting; respectful; trusting; and conducive to questions, divergent thinking, and feedback. All learners must be able to freely express their feelings and thoughts. Learning and achieving learning objectives are facilitated when learners are listened to in a respectful and open manner.

Chapter 3: Implement Health Education

Introduction to Implementation

Implementation is a critical part of the health educator's career and responsibilities. It involves the entire start-to-finish process of enacting a health education program. All of the planning, theory, research, and preparation of program design become reality when implementing an intervention. From building an appropriate plan of action to conducting the final portion of the program evaluation, implementation is where the "rubber meets the road." Health educators must be prepared to push a program from idea to reality, and implementation strategies are the tools for success.

On the CHES Examination, program implementation accounts for only one of seven official sections, and it is the area that typically includes the most questions and is reflected most heavily in the final score. Health program implementation unites the theoretical and practical responsibilities of the health educator. Skills and knowledge of program implementation are essential to successfully executing a health education class, campaign, public health initiative, advocacy endeavor, and other practical applications of health education and health promotion. A thorough understanding of program implementation will allow health educators to more easily conduct successful programs, gain recognition for well-designed programs, and evaluate interventions in a meaningful way. Furthermore, publishing program experiences often depends on properly implementing a well-designed intervention.

The surest way to succeed as a health educator is to become skilled at start-to-finish program implementation. Use the concepts described below as a starting point for a thorough study of implementation.

Plan of Action

An **action plan** or **plan of action** is essential to developing, implementing, and evaluating a health program. Although the term indicates its general meaning, an action plan is usually a written directive documenting the health educator's intentions for each program stage. The plan should be entirely completed (including a plan for program evaluation) prior to implementing the program with participants. The plan should be updated regularly as changes are made to the expected program, its objectives, and any relevant processes connected to it. A plan of action can serve as a guide and motivator for keeping the program on track.

Health Status Evaluation/Community Needs Assessment
Prior to implementing a health program, the health educator must conduct a health status evaluation of the target population. This evaluation is called a **community needs assessment** or, simply, a needs assessment. Needs assessments gather and analyze data about population priorities and health status. This assessment is essential to the program planning process and must be conducted before designing a program. In some program planning models, community involvement in a needs assessment will

direct program design. Community members often request an intervention to address their concerns. While health educators must always remember the importance of community support, they must also use their leadership skills to build consensus for addressing a community need that is demonstrated by data and that meets the SMART (specific, measurable, attainable, realistic, and timely) criteria.

Needs assessments help health educators identify a specific health need for a particular population segment. The creation of needs assessments is easier when these two influences are present: (1) appropriate data sources and (2) community involvement.

Baseline Data Collection
Typically, health educators have funding or organizational guidance, requiring a health program focused on a particular topic or a specific population. Health educators rarely have the opportunity to select a health program topic that appeals to them. Regardless of whether a narrow topic is already selected, **baseline data collection** is necessary for program planning and successful program implementation. This collection requires the health educator to gather information about important health issues, population characteristics, program techniques, and potential implementation methods. The health educator can use this baseline data collection to better understand the targeted health issue and priority population by exploring information about disease processes, population risks, and potential disease or population attributes that may be amenable to change.

Baseline data collection can completed using primary or secondary sources. **Primary data collection** involves interviews, focus groups, and/or surveys administered by the health educator. These techniques can be time-consuming and costly, but may offer invaluable qualitative and quantitative information about the target population. These methods may be particularly useful to determine whether a particular program idea will appeal to members of the target population.

Secondary data is often accessible, comprehensive, and informative quantitative information. Large data sets, such as the National Health and Nutrition Examination Survey (NHANES, http://www.cdc.gov/nchs/nhanes.htm), Census Data (http://www.census.gov/2010census/data/), and the National Youth Risk Behavior Survey (YRBS, http://www.cdc.gov/HealthyYouth/yrbs/data/), are readily available to the public and can help health educators determine potential program topics. Data sets are commonly used to help educators understand the prevalence of a health problem, demographics of a target population, and morbidity and mortality rates linked to the health problem. Although secondary data sets can offer a wealth of information, they often lack detailed information about small subsets of populations that may be targeted by a particular program. For example, information about family planning habits among the Somali population in Columbus, Ohio may be essentially nonexistent in secondary data sets; in this case, primary data collection may be a health educator's only option to better understand the baseline needs of the target population. All health educators should be familiar with common datasets that may be useful in their primary fields of focus.

Regardless of the type of data collected by the health educator, the relevance and quality of the information is essential. Health educators should search for or collect data that is unbiased, valid, reliable, and appropriate for the targeted population. Academic journals; government surveys and websites; and peer-reviewed, validated tools are excellent starting points for baseline data collection. Primary data collection should also be carefully designed to avoid misleading, biased, or incomplete results.

Community Involvement
Some health programs revolve entirely around the needs and desires expressed by community members participating in a community needs assessment. Other programs are designed in advance and then pitched to community members to win their support afterward. Typically, health educators benefit from community and stakeholder involvement as early as possible in the program planning process. Involving key community leaders, organizations, and relevant individuals required for program success can ease program design and implementation.

Health educators should consider creating a program committee to facilitate planning, implementing, and evaluating the program. Committee members can promote the program and improve the possibility for success. For a long-term program, committees can help establish a structure for program survival and transition. Although committees can help significantly with program implementation, group dynamics and competing interests may sometimes complicate progress and impede program success; proper guidance from the health educator can be essential to avoiding or resolving committee disagreements.

Involving individuals can help health educators design a feasible and relevant program for a target population. Additionally, initial stakeholder involvement and support can make it easier to obtain funding, licenses, and other essential resources for program implementation. Some health education efforts will require various levels of reliance on community groups and organizations to achieve program goals. Four descriptions of potential relationships include networking, coordinating, cooperating, and collaborating.

Networking, the lowest level of community interaction, is where the health educator simply communicates and exchanges mutually beneficial information with other groups. Networking can help the health educator better understand the environment or context in which the program will be implemented, but no further assistance is usually acquired. **Coordinating** goes one step further than networking to offer feedback between the health programmers and the group or organization; both sides may modify activities (such as scheduled class times) to accommodate the other group and their shared goals. **Cooperating** involves exchanging information, coordinating activities, and sharing resources (such as staff or facilities). **Collaborating** is the most interdependent and profound relationship of the four. It involves all of the above levels of interaction as well as the attempt to improve each other's abilities to achieve shared goals. In many ways, collaboration is a partnership of shared risks and rewards of program implementation. At each of these progressive levels, the health educator may be working with multiple groups or organizations; the level of desired interaction with each group may vary.

Timeline, Objectives, and Resources
No plan of action is complete without an overarching layout of the program's expected timeline, primary and secondary goals and objectives, and necessary resources. Although all of these items are typically modified during the planning and implementation processes, they should be considered as early as possible in the process to provide direction, to enable communication of the general plan, and to guide the educator and committee members in resource acquisition.

Timelines provide the plan of action with a schedule—a backbone to organize the progression from planning to implementing to evaluating to program termination. They typically include general deadlines for all major events involved in preparing for, conducting, and concluding an intervention. Specific tools for timeline management will be further discussed later.

Action plans should also include a list of specific program **objectives**. Objectives are specific, measurable tasks for completing every aspect of the program. They include administrative or process objectives (such as hiring staff or printing fliers), learning objectives (such as improving participants' understanding of a disease prevention technique), behavioral or action objectives (such as increasing the number of cardiovascular sessions to twice weekly for at least half of all participants), environmental objectives (such as cleaning a park), and program or outcome objectives (such as preventing 50 cases of infection). Not all programs will include every type of objective.

Objectives offer staff involved with program implementation a specific list of measurable endpoints for each program task. They provide specific task guidelines that must be completed before, during, and after an intervention to enable program success; completing objectives should result in achieving program goals. Each objective should serve as a criterion for program evaluation.

Resources cover a wide range of necessary items, monies, staff, facilities, and plans the health educator must have in place to conduct an intervention. The action plan should acknowledge and list, in as much detail as possible, the anticipated resource needs. Once objectives are written, it is usually easier to estimate the number of staff members, type of locations, variety of advertisement streams, assortment of supporting organizations, and amount of funds that will be required to meet the objectives. Having a list of available, necessary resources before implementing the program will enable the health educator to plan appropriately for program promotion and resource acquisition. It will also increase the chance for a smooth program implementation process.

Pretesting

Pretesting is a critical part of the planning and implementation processes of health education interventions. It allows health education specialists to better predict the program's success and to evaluate the program's effectiveness in a formal manner.

There are two types of **pretesting**. The first tests specific program features and/or intervention with members of the target population before officially launching the program; this type of pretest resembles pilot testing, but evaluates only a small portion of the total program. **Pilot testing** may include a test run of the entire program with a smaller number of participants; piloting allows the health educator to test program processes and improve (or abandon) the program before full implementation. Pilot testing is discussed more in-depth later in this chapter. The second type of pretesting involves collecting baseline data on the target population, before program implementation, to compare with post-test data collected after the program is completed.

Pretests should be carefully designed and structured to offer the most useful information possible to the health educator. For example, a carefully designed pretest of a recipe for a healthy cooking class with members of the priority population may give the educator critical information about the cultural appropriateness of particular ingredients. If pretest participants are asked for feedback and feel comfortable responding honestly, problems can be corrected before launching the full program. In this way, a program can avoid considerable difficulties during full-fledged implementation.

In pretesting designed to collect information about the population before the intervention's education portion begins, the pretest should ideally be based on evidence or existing tools. Health educators have a responsibility to program participants not to overburden them with useless or cumbersome data collection. Data collection tools should collect only information directly relevant to the intervention that will be used to evaluate the program's effectiveness. Furthermore, pretests should be designed according to the program's theories and models. For example, if a program is designed to affect change based on the Health-Belief Model, reasonable pretest questions could assess the threat of a health problem as perceived by participants. After the program has been completed, the post-test would assess the new perceived threat reported by participants to help the health educator determine if the program successfully changed that metric.

NOTE: Any pretest of this nature should be carefully designed to assess its appropriateness; cultural issues, health literacy, native language, age, and other characteristics of the priority population will affect pretest design. Pretests can be administered via interviews, written exams, digital polling, web surveys, and many other methods—just ensure the method corresponds well to the needs and comfort level of your priority population.

The Intervention Process

All health programs involve an **intervention**—a treatment or experience to which the target population will be exposed. All interventions should be based on strategies supported by data, research, and theory. There may be considerable work involved with non-intervention portions of a health program, but interventions are the primary point at which participants will interact with the health educator's program. As such, interventions are a crucial portion of program implementation. They must be carefully planned, responsibly implemented, and thoughtfully evaluated.

Interventions may take several forms. Depending on the nature of the health issue being addressed, the availability of resources, and the key characteristics of the target population, a program's intervention will consist of different activities. Based on initial data collection, community and stakeholder consultation, established theory and program models, and published research from similar populations, the health educator may determine that certain intervention methods are more likely than others to be successful. Common options for intervention activities include a focus on advocacy or policy, behavioral, communication or educational, community mobilization, environmental, or service. In addition to choosing the type of intervention activity, the health educator must also determine the best ways to introduce, administer, and evaluate the intervention.

Advocacy and **policy interventions** target large-scale changes in political environments or written organizational or governmental policies. Advocacy activities for an intervention could include coalition-building or creating a letter-writing campaign advocating a particular change. Advocacy interventions may also include media and community outreach to have others notice an issue affecting the targeted population (for example, an intervention may advertise and sponsor a race or march to raise awareness about child hunger in the community). Policy interventions may include activities like lobbying a governmental or organizational board on behalf of the target population or crafting new legislation. For example, health policy interventions may try to draft and gain acceptance for a clean water resolution, youth curfews, a tax increase on cigarettes, or automobile emission restrictions. In organizations, policy interventions may work with the company board to implement a policy supporting breaks for breastfeeding mothers or gym membership reimbursements for staff.

A **behavioral intervention** will be designed to impact the actions of participants. For example, the health educator may design a peer intervention aimed at helping participants eliminate tobacco use. Activities in a behavioral intervention will be geared toward promoting, enabling, and sustaining a behavioral change in participants. Although behavior has complex roots, sustained behavioral modification is possible with carefully planned and implemented interventions and willing, committed participants. Behavioral interventions can be extremely effective, but may require multiple sessions, certified trainers, and considerable financial resources.

A **communication** or **educational intervention** may consist entirely of information distributed through one or more channels. Communication activities are part of every intervention, but some interventions are composed solely of written, spoken, digital, or other media. A common example of a strict communication intervention is a public health campaign via posters placed in doctors' offices promoting vaccination. Communication interventions can reach large numbers of people and may offer comparatively affordable methods for transmitting health-related information to the priority population. However, they typically provide little opportunity to interact with the target population and may not reach all desired participants. They can also be difficult to evaluate. Educational interventions may consist of more than just written or spoken communications. They may include more interactive activities, such as classes, question and answer sessions, support groups, and lectures. Communication and educational interventions may hold behavior change as an ultimate goal, but their actual program objectives typically focus on simple changes in the target population's knowledge, attitudes, and skills.

Community mobilization interventions involve attempts to energize a community to act on its own behalf. Common activities in these types of interventions include campaigns to motivate and organize members of a neighborhood, cultural group, organization, or larger group of people to tackle a health issue affecting their population. These interventions may also involve lobbying, grassroots canvassing, town hall meetings, and media activities promoting changes and commitment to a health issue by members of the community. Community mobilization interventions may seem similar to advocacy programs, but they focus on building community involvement, collaboration, and eventual ownership of the current health issue.

Environmental interventions may target changes in a physical or social environment. Activities can be varied and may or may not involve much direct interaction with the target population. For example, an intervention may involve designing a street plan for safe sidewalks in a run-down neighborhood. Although baseline data collection would involve determining whether the sidewalk is desired or likely to be used by community residents, the actual intervention activity would primarily involve a change to the built environment. Social environment interventions could include activities geared toward reducing barriers to scheduling doctors' appointments for the uninsured or toward improving acceptance of a "culture of safety" among employees for reporting harassment.

Service interventions typically have altruistic aims; they involve activities designed to improve a specific health problem in a target population. For example, the intervention may offer free vaccinations to children in inner-city health clinics or complimentary blood glucose screens to passers-by at a health fair. Service interventions may also have activities with other objectives, such as patient education.

Delivering an Intervention
Depending on the health concern being addressed, in intervention planning, certain types of intervention activities may take priority over others. For example,

interventions targeting a behavioral change may require multiple sessions, while interventions aimed at offering education may be successful after a single meeting. The amount of exposure received by the target population may be referred to as the **dose** of an intervention. The dose also refers to the number of contacted participants, the intervention duration, and the exposure intensity (for example, one-on-one counseling versus a group lecture).

The **delivery method** for the program consists of the strategy and logistics of intervention implementation. Methods chosen for an intervention will depend on available data, program resources, population characteristics, models and theories, and program goals. For example, the size of the target population may demand a mass media communication intervention, the cultural characteristics of the target population may require an informational session in a language other than English, or the health behavior theories and previous programming successes may strongly support the use of activities for a text message support intervention. The health educator will have to consider all factors identified during the needs assessment, action plan creation, community and stakeholder consultation, and further research to determine the best mode of intervention delivery. He/she must determine where, when, how frequently, and in what way to deliver the planned activities.

Intervention Strategy
After the plan of action has been designed and program objectives have been developed, the intervention can be established in detail. The health educator must conduct considerable research and remember available resources when determining what type of intervention to use for a health program. The strategy selected for the program will depend on the nature of the health problem, the type of objectives needed to achieve the desired change, and the limitations regarding program resources, reach, and scope. Additionally, theories and models are essential for constructing sound, evidence-based intervention strategies.

Theories and models are essential to successful intervention planning. They offer guidelines for intervention structure and strategy and legitimacy for presenting the program to communities, funding agencies, stakeholders, and peers in the world of research and health education.

A **theory** is, according to the National Cancer Institute, "a systematic way of understanding events or situations. It is a set of concepts, definitions, and propositions that explain or predict these events or situations by illustrating the relationships between variables." [http://www.cancer.gov/cancertopics/cancerlibrary/theory.pdf page 4]. Dozens of theories (some much better and more useful than others) have been developed to explain human behavior, learning, and decision-making.

A **model** is usually a combination of different theoretical constructs designed to help health educators understand the contexts and situations they will face in health education and health promotion programs. Multiple program planning and implementation models exist, but not all will be equally applicable for the type of program you may need to build. Health educators should select a model that will help them accomplish program goals, but they should also acknowledge that rarely does a single theory or model, on its own, perfectly design and implement an intervention.

Many health education interventions use multiple theories or models (or parts thereof) to address the unique aspects of the chosen health issue and target population. Some of the most common theories and models used in health education intervention planning and implementation are described below.

- **Health-Belief Model.** This popular model explains individual health behaviors by emphasizing the importance of health beliefs and attitudes. Implementing an intervention based on an understanding of this model typically involves addressing the model's concepts with educational or behavioral interventions. Concepts include perceived susceptibility, perceived severity, perceived benefits, perceived barriers, cues to action, and self-efficacy. For example, an intervention may attempt to reduce participants' perceived barriers to obtaining health insurance by explaining and helping them complete the necessary paperwork.

- **Theory of Reasoned Action (Theory of Planned Behavior).** This theory argues that behavior is influenced by an individual's intention to act. This intention to act is built on several contributing concepts: behavioral beliefs and the person's attitude toward a behavior, normative beliefs and the subjective norm, and control beliefs and perceived behavioral control. Interventions following this theory may aim to foster beliefs that produce a favorable idea of behavior and encourage creating an intention to act. For example, a communication campaign encouraging HIV testing may target normative beliefs by playing commercials showing people representative of the target population discussing their positive experiences in seeking testing.

- **Stimulus Response Theory.** This classic psychological theory describes behavior as a reaction to an event or incentive. It relies on the idea that people can be conditioned, by incentive or reinforcement, to act certain ways. An intervention following this theory might try to change the participants' response to a stimulus (perhaps by teaching stress relief techniques to avoid smoking when around other smokers) or to reinforcement for performing a certain health behavior (perhaps by emphasizing increased energy levels instead of grocery bills when on a balanced diet).

- **Elaboration Likelihood Model (ELM).** This model attempts to explain how people process and internalize communications (such as persuasive messages, television commercials, etc.). Programs that rely heavily on a single contact with participants or that offer only communication interventions may use this model. For example, a health educator may consider the ELM and carefully design a radio announcement to increase the chances that the target audience will change its attitude toward flu shots.

- **Precaution Adoption Process Model (PAPM).** This model describes a variety of stages along an individual's path to action. Regarding any health issue or action, participants may be unaware, unengaged, or undecided. Then, participants may decide to act or not act. Once a participant has decided to act, he/she may act and maintain the behavior. Depending on the stage of a program's participants, an intervention may use different strategies to move them along the continuum from lack of awareness to long-term maintenance of a health behavior. For example, if participants have already decided to lose weight, a health education program may offer techniques for starting an exercise regimen and maintaining it for six months.

- **Transtheoretical Model/Stages of Change.** This model offers another description of the pathway to action for health behaviors. Much like PAPM, the Stages of Change include pre-contemplation, contemplation, preparation to act, action, maintenance, and termination of the behavior. At any point in the process, participants can relapse to a prior stage. An intervention based on this model may try to move pre-contemplative members of the target population into the contemplation or preparation stages by offering informational brochures and/or a free session with a general health counselor. The **Community Readiness Model** involves similar stages of change for groups, organizations, and communities, but requires consideration of group dynamics for program strategy implementation.

- **Social Cognitive Theory.** This broad theory predicts behavior results from both involuntary responses to stimuli and learned attitudes and abilities. Concepts in this theory typically include reciprocal determinism, behavioral capability, reinforcements, expectations, expectancies, self-control and self-efficacy, and coping abilities. An intervention based on social cognitive theory could train program participants to interpret nutrition labels to improve self-efficacy levels.

- **Diffusion of Innovations Theory.** This theory describes the way innovations (products or ideas) are accepted by a population. Innovators and early adopters will begin using a product before the early majority, late majority, and laggards. Many interventions may use this theory to define their target population and select appropriate strategies. For instance, effective encouragement for innovators may involve promoting the "trailblazer" mentality, while encouraging laggards to adopt a new health behavior may involve social norming messaging.

- **PRECEDE-PROCEED.** This theory is a very popular program planning model that helps health educators address a wide variety of constructs while planning and implementing an intervention. It covers predisposing, reinforcing, and enabling constructs in ecological diagnosis and evaluation as well as policy, regulatory, and organizational constructs in educational and environmental development. By researching and addressing the constructs presented in this model, health educators can be better prepared to implement a program that adequately addresses the target population's needs.

- **The Logic Model.** This popular program planning and evaluation model offers users a way to visualize and organize a program's inputs, outputs, and outcomes {see http://www.uiweb.uidaho.edu/extension/LogicModel.pdf}. **Inputs** in the model include anything the health educator or program sponsor invests in the program to implement it. Time, money, staff, facilities, and community partners are all considered program inputs. The program's activities, materials, and participants constitute a program's **outputs**. By manipulating inputs and outputs, the program aims to achieve its **outcomes**: short-term and medium-term changes in behaviors, skills, attitudes, knowledge along with other targets of program objectives. Long-term outcomes often include larger-scale changes in policy or environment. This model encourages health educators to always consider context when implementing an intervention, including any **external factors** (such as competing programs, news coverage of a related topic, and funding opportunities) that may influence successful implementation. Logic models should help health educators identify the **assumptions** on which they are basing program implementation. For example, anticipating a long-term outcome of reduced homelessness rates indicates an assumption that the program can modify certain factors to prevent or reverse homelessness.

Every theory and model has limitations. The health educator must be able to connect concepts of theories and guidelines of models to the target population's needs. Additionally, theories and models must be considered in their intended contexts. Concepts designed to explain and predict intra- and interpersonal behavior are often very different from those designed to explain community behavior. Applying theories and models appropriately can aid planning and effective implementation of health education programs.

Cultural Competence
In addition to considering the structure and strategy behind an intervention, the health educator must note how the target population receives the intervention. **Cultural competence** is the ability to understand, recognize, respect, and appropriately respond to the variety of social mores, attitudes, values, beliefs, and behaviors that characterize a group of people. It requires the health educator to understand and accommodate the target population's cultural characteristics that may impact the intervention's effectiveness. By preparing in advance and responding appropriately to issues as they arise, health educators and those involved in implementing the intervention can confidently address the unique cultural needs of the target population.

In addition to the typical cultural issues a health educator must research, an intervention strategy must also consider the target population's **health literacy**. Health literacy is not simply the ability to read and write; it also includes the ability to comprehend information in the context of health and healthcare. Health literacy acknowledges an individual's situation (a routine care visit versus a cancer biopsy visit), his/her physical location (home versus an intensive care unit), an individual's social and cultural characteristics (including language, religious beliefs, and familial relationships), and an individual's contextual influences (such as education, numeracy skills, and even the presence of a patient and relatable physician) on his/her capacity to process health-related information. All of these factors will contribute to and influence an individual's health literacy skills. A target population's general health literacy will influence the sophistication level of a health educator's communication. [http://www.nap.edu/openbook.php?record_id=10883&page=32]

Regardless of the anticipated health literacy level or language barriers of the target population, the vast majority of health interventions should be administered in **plain language**. Extensive education does not necessarily mean someone has good health literacy skills. Plain language is intended to be simple enough for people to understand, interpret, and act on—without needing others' assistance. Plain language typically uses simple explanations of health concepts, avoids medical jargon (or defines complex terms in basic language), and provides essential information in small, readable chunks. Many documents that use plain language will also prioritize the most important points and consider organization, leaving plenty of white space or using graphics to help illustrate a point. Health educators should strive to use plain language in all consent forms, program advertisements, informational brochures, and health education materials (including PowerPoint presentations) used for programs. [http://www.health.gov/communication/literacy/plainlanguage/PlainLanguage.htm]

In addition to addressing literacy and language concerns, messages included in a health education intervention should be designed while considering the particular target population. The health educator must consider the age, education level, cultural background, attitudes, skills, motivation, disease status, and other characteristics when crafting health education messages and materials. For example, a group of sexually active teenagers will respond to different messaging strategies than college students, just as a population of diabetic Mexican immigrants will respond to different messaging strategies than diabetic senior citizen African Americans.

The amount of information known about the target population, as well as the number of resources available for creating intervention message materials, will determine how much a message can be tailored or targeted. **Tailored messages** involve using individual-level information regarding needs, preferences, beliefs, and attitudes to develop personalized interventions. This information is often gathered from pretests and can be used to create a message or intervention more relevant to a particular participant. **Targeted messages** involve using group-level shared characteristics to develop specific intervention activities. This information may be gathered through initial data collection on the target population or through a pretest of the participants. Targeted messages and interventions often consider cultural beliefs, attitudes, values, and demographics to make the information as accessible and engaging as possible.

Implementation

Implementing a health education program involves enacting program plans, objectives, activities, and evaluations. Furthermore, it executes the administrative, policy and regulatory, monitoring, and resource use aspects of the health education program detailed in the action plan. Without implementing health education, interventions would not occur; plans would remain unfinished, target populations would remain unreached, and health problems would remain unaddressed.

Five Phases of Implementation
In the field of health education programming, many experts acknowledge at least some variation of McKenzie, Neiger, and Thackeray's Five Phases of Implementation: (1) adopt the program, (2) identify and prioritize the tasks to be completed, (3) establish a management system, (4) enact the plans, and (5) end or sustain a program.

Phase One: Adopt the Program
This phase focuses on concepts in program planning and design. It includes identifying and organizing committees, researching and selecting theories and models, and properly preparing to reach the target audience (data collection, marketing, and consultation). After adopting and establishing a program idea, the health educator proceeds to the next phase of implementation.

Phase Two: Identify and Prioritize Tasks
When creating an in-depth plan of action, health programmers must consider all duties—large and small—that must be performed to bring the program to fruition. Creating program objectives can help establish a detailed list of necessary tasks. To appropriately prioritize these tasks, the health educator must know in what order the tasks must be completed to ensure successful program implementation and completion.

Establishing tools for task lists and organization can help the educator, other program staff members, and community committee members to understand the process and keep the intervention on track for success. Tools, such as basic timelines, Gantt charts, PERT, and CPM, can help health educators and program contributors successfully implement the intervention.

Timelines and **task development timelines** list the tasks that must be completed along with their time frames for completion. They are simple graphics or lists that convey the most basic task information; the health educator can mark a check or an "X" by a completed task to visually indicate progress.

Public Domain (with restrictions) Image:
http://commons.wikimedia.org/wiki/File:Program_timeline.png

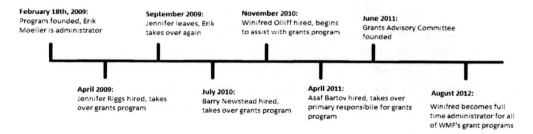

Gantt charts, named after their creator Henry Gantt, offer a more visual indication of what task must be completed, the time frame for its completion , and the progress toward that completion (marked by a partial, thin line underneath the full, thick line indicating the expected task duration or by using multiple colors and color-coding). In both regular timelines and Gantt charts, sections of the tasks can be separated or coded by the person responsible for them, allowing users to see how their tasks overlap or coordinate with those of others.

Public Domain Gantt Chart Image:
http://commons.wikimedia.org/wiki/File:Gantt_Chart_10-21.JPG

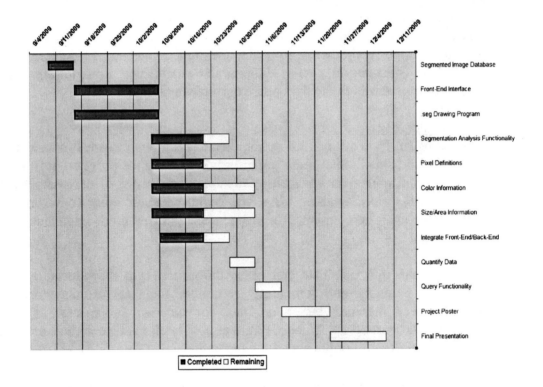

The **Program Evaluation and Review Technique (PERT)** is a popular project management tool in many fields. It is designed to ease complex task and schedule management through a combination of simple visuals and basic task information. A diagram of each task shows a graphic representation of the order and duration of tasks, showing viewers which tasks must be completed before other tasks can begin and how long a task is expected to last. This tool is similar in appearance to the **Critical Path Method (CPM)**. CPM diagrams tasks with completion times in a similar network organization to PERT, but requires the identification of a *critical path*: the particular tasks that cannot be delayed without delaying the entire project. Other tasks have slack, or some flexibility, in their time frames for completion. This allows users to prioritize the order and importance of key tasks to keep the program on schedule. PERT and CPM both have considerably more details for their full use and can be studied in-depth in the project or process management literature.

Phase Three: Establish a Management System

For any program to be successfully implemented, the health educator or program manager must be able to make decisions about the method of management, the use of resources, and the degree of management required for the program. For example, does the program require constant oversight by multiple managers, or will a part-time staff member suffice? What regulations and ethical standards will affect program implementation and management? Who will be responsible for distributing program resources, and how will program funding be dispersed? The health educator must establish a plan for organizing and responding to all program concerns regarding intervention implementation.

Phase Four: Enact the Plans

If the action plan is ever to become a real intervention, it must be implemented. Depending on the nature and duration of the program, the health educator may wish to implement it all at once, in phases, or in a pilot test. For one-shot programs like health fairs, implementing the entire program all at once may be the only practical option. Many programs, however, may benefit from partial implementation or pilot testing. By implementing in phases (for example, beginning a vaccination promotion program at three clinics before phasing it into a total of twelve), the health educator allows for unique evaluation opportunities as well as program improvement or adjustment before full-fledged implementation. Similarly, **pilot testing** serves as a field test or practice run designed to test the program before fully implementing it. This trial run allows the health educator to evaluate and adjust the small version of the program before committing all of the required time and resources to implementing the complete action plan. A pilot test should be performed with a group as similar as possible to members of the target population to avoid misleading results. Pilot testing is most useful if feedback is collected and incorporated into an improved program design before launching the full version.

Phase Five: End or Sustain the Program

If a program has been put into action, the health educator must be able to define some sort of end point. Will the program continue until it has accomplished all goals and objectives? Will the program run indefinitely as a general benefit to the community? How long will funding, staff, and community interest enable the program's survival? How will resources be managed if the program is to be sustained or transferred to the supervision of another entity? Before the program is implemented, the health educator must plan, in detail, the program's termination or maintenance.

Health educators may face strict requirements or difficult decisions if programs do not yield results in the planned timeline or if resource limitations prevent the envisioned program duration from becoming reality. Some programs must follow a certain schedule regardless of success, while others may have potential for institutionalization, maintenance by an alternative organization, program revision, or the receipt of additional resources (such as grant money or volunteer staff).

Evaluations must be completed to determine the program's progress and impact, and resources must be handled appropriately to ensure a smooth conclusion to the endeavor.

The Ethics of Implementation

Ethics are a critical part of planning, implementing, and evaluating health education programs. Without understanding essential ethical guidelines and expectations, health educators may inadvertently commit ethical blunders that can leave them or their organizations susceptible to significant legal or reputational repercussions. In addition to understanding the NCHEC Health Education Code of Ethics (http://www.nchec.org/credentialing/docs/nch-mr-tab3-113.htm), health educators must understand what constitutes ethical program implementation and recognize common errors in ethical behavior.

Health educators will undoubtedly face ethical decisions and dilemmas during their careers. Although many ethical quandaries can be avoided with careful planning and conscientious program implementation, health educators must know how to deal with difficult ethical situations if they arise. Some key concepts and principles are discussed below.

Many health educators recognize the **Belmont Report** of 1979 (http://www.hhs.gov/ohrp/humansubjects/guidance/belmont.html) as the critical document providing ethical guidance to anyone working with human populations for research, education, and or formal intervention. The primary ethical principles described by the Belmont Report include respect for persons, beneficence, and justice. Each of these areas must be incorporated into every aspect of interventions with human subjects, often applied through informed consent, risk-benefit assessments, and appropriate selection of participants.

Respect for persons acknowledges individual autonomy and the fact that humans deserve protection. When implementing health education endeavors, the health educator must never forget that participants have a right to make their own decisions about their health and bodies; they deserve to be informed and aware of any potential risks of program participation. In practice, many health education programs require a signature of **informed consent** indicating the participant has received a complete explanation of the program, its **risks and benefits**, and the opportunity to withdraw at any time without fear of retaliation. No person can be forced to participate in an intervention without the entity implementing the intervention crossing an ethical (and sometimes legal) boundary. It is important to note that some benefits may be disproportionate to risks incurred through participation; this inequality may also be considered unethical, as it may cloud decision-making for potential participants (for instance, offering $500 for a blood donation may attract economically disadvantaged participants who would not participate except for the large financial incentive). Informed consent must usually be signed only when the participant or his/her legal guardian completely understand the agreement. Finally, informed consent documents must be written at a language level that is accessible to the participant.

Beneficence requires that intervention participants be treated in a manner that attempts to improve their well-being. At the very least, health educators and other interventionists are expected to adhere to non-maleficence—they must not harm program participants. Any possibility of harm must be disclosed to participants, and participants must be allowed to discontinue their participation at any time. When implementing health education programs, beneficence extends to the **selection of subjects** for programs *as well as for trials and pilot tests*. It is unethical to burden program participants or test subjects without offering a meaningful benefit or compensation. Certain populations are considered vulnerable because of their accessibility or societal positions (prisoners, school children, etc.); any programs targeted at this population must have ethical reasons beyond ease of inclusion for selecting these participants. Furthermore, it may be unethical to select certain participants for the program while excluding others. For example, it may be unethical to select only one race of participants for a program at a health clinic if the health issue also affects members of other races.

Health educators can improve the ethical merit of their interventions by obtaining the approval of an **Institutional Review Board** or IRB. These committees are often stationed in hospitals, universities, public health departments, and private organizations to ensure the safety of program participants. IRBs review the ethical nature of programs and will identify potential areas of concern that must be addressed before the program can be implemented. Interventions involving potentially dangerous interaction with participants must provide pre-identified stopping points if the program does not seem to be benefiting participants or if it is harming them. Similarly, an IRB evaluates an intervention to find other program design elements that may lead to unethical acts of omission, commission, or negligence.

Omission means that the health educator or program has excluded something that should have been included or completed. For example, an ethical problem of omission could be simply forgetting to obtain parental permission before implementing a non-curriculum weight management education class at a middle school.

Commission goes a step further than omission to complete an act that, if it violates an ethical principle, should not have been performed. For example, an ethical problem of commission could involve requiring students to attend a program to which their parents refused consent.

Negligence is committed when a person fails to act reasonably. For example, an ethical problem of negligence could occur if a health educator neglects to offer food and drink to program participants despite all-day participation in a closed environment program. In many cases, the health educator can be legally accountable for negligent behavior.

Review of an action plan by an IRB or ethics committee can help the health educator prevent many possible ethical problems. However, some ethical issues will not be anticipated and may be encountered during program implementation. The health educator must be prepared to deal with potential problems in an ethical manner by relying on the NCHEC guidelines for health educators and a firm understanding of common ethical principles for interventions with human subjects.

Four Ps of Marketing

Although health educators should have some knowledge of marketing to help their programs successfully target and reach the priority population, understanding E. Jerome McCarthy's famous Four Ps of Marketing will suffice for many projects. The Four Ps that should always be considered when implementing a health education intervention are product, price, place, and promotion.

Product
Even though an education program or health promotion project may not include the common definition of a "product," the health educator should view the intervention and its materials as a product. It is the service that the health educator offers, and as such, it should be created to address the target population's needs and wants. A health educator could design the cleverest "Safe Sidewalk" community mobilization program in the world, but if the target population is uninterested, the product or project will ultimately fail. The product that the health educator presents to the target population will have a better chance of succeeding if the health educator conducts the recommended community assessments, consultations, research, theory incorporation, and pretesting discussed above.

Price
Although many health education interventions are technically free of charge to participants, the health educator must consider other costs. Time, effort, travel, childcare, embarrassment, frequency, and other factors are incorporated into a participant's idea of cost. The health educator must ensure the price associated with program participation will be outweighed by the apparent benefits or rewards of the program. For programs that do charge a fee or involve a direct monetary cost to users, the health educator must carefully select a price that makes the product accessible to the target population while still conveying the value of the product.

Place
Health educators must determine where and how to provide the product or program to the target audience. Is the location safe and conducive to the completion of the intervention? Is the facility accessible to the priority population in terms of distance, schedule, and comfort level? For instance, a program could be safely and technologically delivered in a hospital classroom, but if participants live 15 miles away, rely on public transportation, work during the times classes are offered, or inherently distrust medical institutions, the place will be disastrous for the intervention. A health educator should evaluate the place and how a program will be delivered to ensure that it considers the needs and desires of participants.

Promotion
Promotion is the primary aspect of marketing that many health educators envision when they think of advertising a program or intervention. It includes all advertisements, materials, publicity, and outreach undertaken on behalf of the program. Before a health education intervention begins, the program must be advertised to the target population in such a way that will entice people to participate. The health educator must know which communication avenues, product or program designs, communication styles, and advertisement methods are most likely to reach and appeal to the priority population. Some populations may respond best to word-of-mouth and poster announcements in community restaurants and grocery stores, while other groups may be most effectively reached by television commercials. Furthermore, some groups may respond to formal or scientific descriptions of the program, while others (such as high school students) may respond to brief messages in slang or casual language. Understanding the best method for promoting the product or intervention to the target population can be essential to program success. Targeting promotion efforts effectively may rely on significant research into the population's characteristics and preferences.

Chapter 4: Developing a Research Plan to Evaluate Education

There are many areas of healthcare education that can and should be evaluated with formal and informal research activities. For example, you could evaluate the structures, processes, and outcomes; you could evaluate individual educational offerings or research your overall educational program; or you could research and evaluate individual educational activities and/or the overall educational program in terms of learner satisfaction, cost avoidance, and other potential benefits such as decreased rates of hospitalization, self-care abilities, and active participation in health promotion and preventive health.

Regardless of what you are researching, the research steps and research plan are essentially the same.

Types of Research

There are two types of research, each of which has different types of data and data analysis: quantitative research and qualitative research.

Quantitative research is more frequently used than qualitative research. At times, people erroneously view quantitative research as scientific and qualitative research as unscientific or "soft science." Both types are scientific and beneficial when generating new knowledge and evaluating educational activities.

Quantitative Research
Quantitative research involves collecting data and using numbers, mathematics, and statistics. It is a valid, systematic, logical, and deductive research approach. The researcher, using the quantitative method, manipulates the independent variable and determines whether or not this manipulation has changed the dependent variable.

Some research designs used for quantitative research include non-experimental, experimental, quasi-experimental, longitudinal, and cross-sectional research. Two examples of quantitative research appropriate for health educators are: research comparing the effectiveness of computer-based education and live education and research evaluating the outcomes of an educational activity in terms of self-care.

Qualitative Research
Contrastingly, qualitative research employs inductive reasoning and is more subjective than quantitative research. There is no manipulation of independent variables and no hypothesis. This form of research searches for the meaning of a phenomenon.

Some research designs used for qualitative research include philosophical, historical, ethnographic, and phenomenological research. Some examples of qualitative research studies appropriate in the arena of health education include the meaning of helplessness among the chronically ill, the meaning of self-agency among those affected with a health-related problem, and a historical study exploring the evolution of health education over time.

Steps of Research and Research Design

The 10 steps of the research process for quantitative research are:

- The Research Problem:
  The research problem is a statement that includes the area of interest the research will address. For example, it may state that the problem is the effectiveness of a particular educational activity.

- The Purpose:
  The purpose is the aim or goal of the research. For example, "The purpose of the research is to examine the relationship between health education and compliance rates."

- The Literature Review:
  Reviewing the literature is time-consuming. This review gives the researcher more information about the topic under study; a deeper understanding of the research topic; and ideas regarding concepts, possible research designs, and sampling techniques, among other things. The sources of these literature reviews are most often found in professional journals.

- The Theoretical, or Conceptual, Framework:
  A conceptual framework, or theory, is selected to give the research activity some grounding and foundation. This framework can be singular or a combination of several conceptual frameworks. For example, if you are modeling the reduction of stress after a self-care educational theory, you may want to consider a theory like Hans Selye's General Adaptation Syndrome relating to stress and how it impacts the body.

- The Hypothesis:
  Simply stated, a hypothesis is an "educated guess" relating to the effect of the independent variable on the dependent variable. All quantitative research studies have a null hypothesis and at least one experimental hypothesis. Hypotheses are not proven; instead, they can be only supported or refuted.

  An example of an experimental hypothesis is, "The outcomes of patient education will improve according to the client's level of participation in all aspects of the planning process." An example of a null hypothesis is, "There will be no differences in terms of outcomes when the client actively participates in all aspects of the planning process."

  Hypotheses are not used in qualitative research.

- Research Design:
  The overall design includes decisions about the interventions or manipulations of the independent variable that will be introduced, the identification of interference or extraneous variables, the timing of data collection, the location of data collection, and the identification of research subjects. Some of these elements, such as variables, are not used for qualitative research.

- Sample Type and Size:
  The members of the sample must be determined and planned. For example, will the sample include both genders and all ages, or will it consist of only males, only females, or only those in a specific age group?

  The sample size must also be determined. Small samples impede successful research, and overly large samples are difficult to manage and collect data from. Some suggest that a major research project should have 100 subjects; others say that fewer subjects are needed. Many studies use at least 30 subjects.

- Instruments and Measurement Tools:
  Instruments and measurement tools are also planned for. Details about these tools are thoroughly discussed in the next section. Measurement tools are used only for quantitative research.

- Data Collection Procedure:
  How will the data be collected? Data can be collected through observation, surveys, and rating scales, among other methods. All data collection, however, must be accurate and unbiased.

- Data Analysis:
  Quantitative data is analyzed with mathematics and statistics. Qualitative data is narrative, so it is analyzed by identifying patterns, trends, and themes throughout the narrative data. Data analysis is discussed further in a later section.

Data Collection Instruments and Tools

Heath educators most often explore and measure physiological, psychological, and social variables. An example of a physiological variable is the vital signs of pulse rate and blood pressure; examples of psychological variables include perceived levels of anxiety, level of depression, and level of self-efficacy and self-care.

Even though many data collection tools can be "home-made," it is preferable to use a standardized data collection and measurement tool that has withstood the rigors of validity and reliability testing.

Validity and Reliability

The best data measurement tools have a high degree of validity and reliability. Validity is defined as a tool's ability to actually measure what it is supposed to measure. For example, if a health educator is researching the relationship between education and levels of wellness, then it is levels of wellness—not another variable such as health seeking—that must be measured.

Reliability is defined as a tool's ability to consistently measure the variable over time with the same results and among different data collectors (inter-rater reliability).

Scales

Measurement Scales

Scales collect quantitative data that relates to the variables of interest. For example, feelings, beliefs, opinions, and other perceptions can be measured mathematically with a scale.

There are several types of scales including:

- Yes/No Scales:
  These scales are dichotomous and, therefore, do not collect the same rich, in-depth data that other scales do. For this reason, they are rarely used.

- Likert Scales:
  These scales are the most commonly used scale. They measure how strongly a statement is agreed to or disagreed to. An example of a Likert Scale item that could be used for health education is:

  The health teaching achieved my personal goals:

1	2	3	4	5
Strongly Disagree	Disagree	Neither Agree nor Disagree	Agree	Strongly Agree

- Guttman Scales:
  This scale ranks choices in terms of the most extreme to the least extreme and vice versa. These scales are especially difficult to develop. It takes a lot of time and skill to develop one that is psychometrically sound.

- Multiple Choice Scales:
  These scales give a fixed set of answers to choose from. The subject can select only one response or multiple responses. To be sound, these scales must be free of ambiguity and have mutually exclusive items. Below is an example of this type of scale.

Your level of education is:

_____ Less than a high school, or secondary school, diploma

_____ High school, or secondary school, diploma

_____ At least 2 years of college

Data Collection Techniques

Some data collection techniques are simple and less costly than others. Additionally, some methods are appropriate for only quantitative or qualitative research or both. Virtually all data collection techniques have distinct advantages and disadvantages.

Researchers consider many factors before determining data collection techniques. Some of these considerations include costs, characteristics and traits of the subjects, amount of time necessary to collect the data, purpose and setting of the research, and the type of research being conducted (quantitative or qualitative).

Some data collection techniques are:
- Observation (direct and indirect)
- Focus groups
- Face-to-face interviews
- Logs
- Questionnaires (mailed and telephonic)
- Diaries and journals
- Documents
- Critical incidents
- Audits

Analysis of Quantitative Data: Statistics and Mathematics

The analysis of quantitative data ranges from the simple to the complex. Mathematics and statistics can be done with pen and pencil, with readily available and accessible software such as Microsoft's Excel, or with sophisticated software such as IBM's Statistical Product and Service Solutions (SPSS).

Descriptive Statistics

There are two basic types of descriptive statistics: measures of central tendency and measures of variability.

Measures of Central Tendency
Measures of central tendency reference quantitative data to a "bell-shaped curve." Statistics that cluster around the center of the bell-shaped curve are the mean, mode, and median. The mean is the average of all of the values, or numbers, in the set of

numbers; the mode is the most frequently occurring number, or score, in the set of numbers; and the median is the middle number in the set of numbers.

Measures of Variability

Measurements of statistical variability include the range, variance, and standard deviation. The range is the difference of the smallest and largest number in the group of numbers. For example, the range of 12 to 22 is 10 (the difference between 22 and 12).

The variance and standard deviation tell the researcher how spread out the data is compared to the bell-shaped curve. Variance shows how much the values vary around the mean; it tells us how far away the numbers are from the mean, or the average. They can be close to the mean or spread out far away from the mean.

The standard deviation is similar to variance. It, too, shows how much variance or dispersion there is around the mean. A low-standard deviation indicates that the data is closely aligned around the mean; a high-standard deviation indicates that the data is spread out more greatly around the mean.

Standard deviation is the square root of the variance, and it indicates the amount of deviation of the numbers away from the mean. Variance is symbolized as S^2. To calculate the standard deviation, find the square root of the variance. Standard deviation is symbolized as S.

Inferential Statistics

Inferential statistics are more complicated than descriptive measurements of central tendency and measurements of variance using statistical methods such as mean, mode, median, range, variance, and standard deviation.

Some basic inferential statistics that you should know are the T-test, Chi-square test, and correlation coefficients.

The T-test and Chi-square test allow us to generalize the research findings to other groups or populations. They indicate if the findings are, or are not, statistically significant. They also indicate if the research results occurred as the result of chance, or accident, or as a result of the manipulation of the independent variable. For example, when the result of the T-test is $p < .02$, it means there is less than a 2% possibility that chance or accident has occurred; the result is primarily related to the research itself at about 98%. Likewise, $p < .10$ indicates that chance is less than 10%; $p < .20$ means that chance accounts for less than 20%, and about 80% of the change is related to the manipulation of the independent variable.

Educational research studies, without any risks, are usually $p < .05$ or $p < .10$. With life threatening studies, a $p < .01$ or less is typically acceptable.

It is almost impossible to prove causality in research, especially when it comes to human subjects. Human subjects are affected by, and influenced with, too many variables that impact research findings. For this reason, correlation, rather than causality, is used in the vast majority of research.

There are two types of correlation: positive and negative. A positive correlation indicates that both the independent and dependent variables increased or decreased. A negative correlation indicates that one of the variables increased and the other decreased. An example of a positive correlation is increased compliance with an exercise regimen after health education (both increased). An example of a negative correlation is decreased rate of cigarette smoking while continuous social support is given to the client (decreased cigarette smoking; increased social support).

Some other inferential statistics are linear regression, regression analysis, analysis of variance (ANOVA), analysis of covariance (ANCOVA), and factor analysis.

Analysis of Qualitative Data

The analysis of qualitative data is different from the analysis of quantitative data simply because the data is different. Qualitative data is narrative, not numerical. Statistics and mathematical analysis, therefore, are not performed; instead, qualitative data is carefully analyzed for themes, patterns, and trends instead of statistics and mathematics.

All data is read and organized into categories, themes, patterns, content, and key points. As stated previously, qualitative research is inductive rather than deductive. The data, therefore, is analyzed using inductive thinking and logic. The researcher hopes to discover an in-depth knowledge or description of the studied phenomenon by connecting the data in a comprehensive manner, like pieces of a puzzle. For example, if you are interested in the meaning and definition of health, you may want to perform an ethnographic or phenomenological study using interviews.

After you have analyzed all the verbal data, you may understand that health has many meanings including physical rigor and role fulfillment. These definitions of health were inductively determined with inductive reasoning because you discovered these patterns and trends in your narrative interview data. You have moved from the general concept of health to specifics such as physical rigor and role fulfillment.

Interpreting the Evaluation/Research

Before using and applying research to practice, the research must be critiqued and scrutinized to determine if it is sound.

All research has strengths and weaknesses. A thorough critique of research includes all the steps of a research project and all the elements of a research report. These steps and areas of consideration for the research critique are:

- Title
- Abstract
- Introduction
- Review of the literature
- Methodology
- Data analysis
- Discussion of the research findings
- Summary
- Conclusion
- Implications
- Recommendations
- Ethical considerations
- Biases

General Considerations
- Is the research study complete, objective, concise, and presented in an understandable and logical manner?
- Are the tables, charts, and graphs labeled and understandable?
- Are the references appropriate and current?
- Is the research study significant in terms of health education?
- What are the overall strengths of the research project?
- What are the overall weaknesses of the research project?
- Are the findings valid and useful to health educators?
- Are the author's claims substantiated?

Critiquing Quantitative Research

- Title:
  - Is the title brief?
  - Does the title accurately reflect the study and the purpose of the study?
  - Does it reflect the variables and the population?

- Abstract:
  - Does the abstract reflect the purpose of the study and its significance?
  - Does it include the research methodology and information about the sample and sample selection process?
  - Does the abstract include the conclusions and interpretations of the findings?

- Introduction:
  - Is the purpose of the study clearly identified?
  - Is the problem statement included in the introduction?
  - Is the significance of the study included in the introduction?
  - What is the significance of the study?
  - What possible benefits can be derived from this study?

- Are operational definitions included?
- Are the assumptions and delimitations stated?
- Does the introduction reflect possible practical applications?
- Is the hypothesis, or hypotheses, included in the introduction?
- Are the conceptual framework and its appropriateness included in the introduction?
- Is the introduction brief, logical, and understandable?

- Review of Literature:
  - Are all relevant sources included?
  - Unless historically valuable, are the sources current (less than 5 years old)?
  - Are primary sources used when appropriate?
  - Are empirical research studies included?
  - Did it give you in-depth information and a fuller understanding of the topic of interest?
  - Did the researcher obtain and relate information about the study design in terms of methodology, variables, concepts, subjects, sampling, and data analysis, among other things?
  - Is it organized, objective, and without bias?
  - Is the bibliography or reference list complete and appropriate?
  - Is there a reference for every citation in the text?

- Methodology:
  - Is the research design (methodology) clearly identified?
  - Was this methodology appropriate for this research study?
  - Does it detail how the study was conducted?
  - Does it clearly state how the data was analyzed?
  - Was the data analyzed in an appropriate and accurate manner?
  - Is the setting for the research clearly stated and appropriate for the study?
  - Is the type of sample appropriate for this research study?
  - Is this method of sampling appropriate for this research study?
  - Was the sample large enough for the study?
  - Were the subjects representative of the population?
  - Were criteria for inclusion and exclusion of subjects stated and valid?
  - Did the research study clearly indicate what kind or method of measurement and measurement tools were used?
  - Did it include a copy of the measurement instrument that was used?
  - Did the research study include statements about the validity and reliability of the measurement instrument that was used?
  - Was the validity of this instrument sufficient for the study?
  - Was the reliability of this instrument sufficient for the study?
  - Are the data collection methods or interventions used for the study clearly stated and sound?
  - Is the data collection organized?
  - Is the procedure for the data collection methods or interventions clearly stated?

- Data Analysis:
  - What type of data analysis was used?
  - Is the statistical analysis method appropriate for the data and the study?
  - Was the analysis mathematically accurate?
  - Did the analysis support or refute the alternative hypothesis or hypotheses?

- Discussion of the Research Findings:
  - Is the presentation and interpretation of the research findings logical, organized, and cogent?
  - Is the discussion of the research findings complete?
  - Does the discussion of the research findings address cautions relating to generalizing the findings to other populations?

- Summary:
  - Is the summary brief and concise?
  - Does the summary include a brief statement about the purpose of the study?
  - Does the summary include a brief statement about assumptions that underlie the study?
  - Does the summary include a brief statement about the how the hypotheses were tested?
  - What other things should have been included in the summary, but were not?

- Conclusions:
  - Are the conclusions summarized in a logical, brief, and cogent manner?
  - Is the summary of data analysis relating to the null hypothesis and other hypotheses presented in a complete, accurate, and understandable manner?

- Implications of the Study:
  - Do the implications relate to and benefit health education?
  - Is there an emphasis on the importance of this study?

- Recommendations:
  - Are the recommendations consistent with the results of the research findings?
  - Based on the research study, are these recommendations valid and accurate?

- Ethical Considerations:
  - Were all ethical rights and principles upheld?

- Bias:
  - Were sample selection, measurement, response, procedural, and researcher bias present and acknowledged by the researchers?

Critiquing Qualitative Research

The method of critiquing a qualitative research project includes:

1. Philosophical or Theoretical Soundness:
   - Are the findings developed and clearly expressed?
   - Are the findings logically consistent and compatible with the knowledge base of health education?
   - Are the assumptions and methodological procedures consistent and compatible with the philosophical or theoretical basis of the study?
   - Are the data analytic approaches and data interpretation consistent and compatible with the philosophical or theoretical basis of the study?

2. Methodological Consistency and Congruence:
   - Is there adequate documentation supporting the rationale for selection of the participants, context, and location of the study?
   - Are any threats to validity acknowledged?
   - Did the researcher scrupulously adhere to the established procedures?

3. Descriptive Vividness:
   - Did the researcher include essential descriptive information in a clear and understandable manner?
   - Are adequate interpretative and analytic skills demonstrated in the description of the phenomenon of interest?

4. Precise Analysis:
   - Does the analysis accurately interpret the data?

5. Precise Interpretation:
   - Did the outcome of the study give meaning to the phenomenon being studied?
   - Did the researcher present a meaningful and precise picture of the phenomenon being studied?

6. Heuristic Relevance:
   - Did the researcher clearly present the phenomenon?
   - Did the researcher clearly present the applicability of the study to health education?
   - Were you able to readily recognize the phenomenon and its connection to you as a health educator and to the profession of health education?
   - What new knowledge was gained as a result of this study?

Below is the step-by-step procedure for critiquing qualitative research. All of the steps for qualitative research are followed EXCEPT those described below.

1. <u>Data Collection</u>:
   - Are the data collection methods used for the study clearly stated?
   - What are the data collection methods?
     - Direct observation without researcher involvement
     - Direct observation with researcher involvement
     - Interviews
     - Surveys
     - Focus groups
   - Are the procedures for the data collection methods clearly stated?
   - Was the duration of data collection appropriate for the research that was done?

2. <u>Data Analysis</u>:
   - What type of data analysis was used?
   - Was the data analyzed accurately and completely?
   - Did the data analysis answer the research question?

Applying Evaluation/Research Findings

Action Research

The application of research finding is often referred to as action research. The goal of applying research to practice is to improve the quality of education and the overall educational program. Action research has merits for health educators. It improves our practice, it can increase our understanding of health education, and it can improve the situation within which we provide this education.

Research should not be conducted or used as a solitary and personal cognitive exercise. Research should be conducted and USED to improve performance and outcomes.

Research gives health educators the opportunity to:
- Explore new ideas and methods
- Test new ideas and methods
- Determine the effectiveness of new methods and approaches to health teaching
- Reflect on their practice
- Assess their practice
- Become a knowledge maker
- Explore different approaches to teaching
- Collaboratively plan changes in practice
- Provide feedback to fellow health educators

The process of action research focuses on nine basic principles:
- Change
- Reflection
- Participation
- Inclusion

- Sharing
- Understanding
- Repetition
- Practice
- Community

Change is the ultimate goal of action research. Research, like education, should translate into practice. Change occurs when a current practice is altered or changed as the result of action research. Action research is not a one-person job; it requires the active collaboration of a team to effectively investigate the problem, formulate where team members currently are, and determine where team members want to be as a result of the action research.

The Look, Think, and Do Cycle
The Look Think and Do Cycle for action research is a simple and practical way of approaching action research and quality assurance and improvement activities within healthcare organizations and institutions.

This ongoing, cyclical process consists of:
- Looking at the current process
- Thinking about the problem or opportunity for improvement
- Thinking about and developing an action plan
- Acting on a new practice and implementation

The last two steps of action research—developing and implementing a new practice— are finished when existing research is being incorporated and applied to the role of the healthcare educator. This task is not completed by the health educator.

Putting Research Findings into Practice

Before putting research findings into practice, the health educator must critique and evaluate the research study, as previously described for both quantitative and qualitative research studies. If the study is deemed appropriate, the findings can, and perhaps should, be put into practice; conversely, if the research is deemed inappropriate, it should not be put into practice.

Planned Change
Putting research findings into practice should be a planned change. Ideally, a group, rather than a sole individual, should be involved in the planned change using sound group process techniques.

Many planned changes cost money. When the potential benefits of the planned change outweigh the costs of the change, it has potential. Some of the details that should be considered for the budget include line budget items such as staff salaries, costs associated with printing, and new software or hardware. A timetable should also be used. Timetables are a valuable, motivating, goal-oriented way to organize the planned change.

After the plan is completed, implementation begins. During implementation, continual monitoring is necessary. After the change has been completely implemented, the outcomes of the change must be measured periodically to determine whether or not the benefits of the change have occurred and also to determine whether the beneficial outcome continues over time.

Chapter 5: Administer and Manage Health Education

Introduction

Administering and managing health education is quite a varied endeavor. It may involve educating individuals, teaching small groups, coordinating educational conferences for both patients and the public, and initiating health prevention campaigns. The overall goal of health education is to increase knowledge and prevention of illness by providing information that will help prevent chronic health issues.

The responsibilities of administering and managing health education involve assessing needs, assets, and capacities for health education. It requires implementation planning that involves evaluation and research related to health education administration and management. It is important to engage in education about all health issues to provide useful information when needed, especially about topics of interest to both patients and the public.

Health education can occur in a variety of settings including insurance companies, medical clinics, foundations, and health associations. Health education can be provided in hospitals; universities and colleges; county, state, and federal government offices; and nursing homes and assisted living places. Those in health education often contribute content and articles to national magazines, health journals, and online publications.

Many in health education hold Master's degrees from colleges offering Public Health programs. The National Commission on Health Education Credentialing (NCHEC) is raising the standards of educator training levels, and individuals can become certified as a health education specialist (CHES). The exam encompasses several areas of responsibilities for health educators and is available on college campuses throughout the United States. Academic eligibility and successful completion of a written exam demonstrates an individual's ongoing dedication and commitment to continuing education.

The Code of Ethics for Health Educators is based on shared values and beliefs about health education. Aiming for the highest possible standards of conduct and encouraging ethical behavior of colleagues is only part of health educators' responsibilities.

The ultimate goal of assessing and managing health education is to educate, promote, improve, and maintain the health of individuals, families, and communities. A health educator is responsible for maintaining professionalism at all times and encouraging ethical conduct among co-workers. Health educators must answer to their employers and must recognize the limits of their professional capabilities, actions, and activities.

Maintaining integrity in the promotion and delivery of health education is the key to respecting the dignity and rights of all the people health educators serve. Plans and policies may need to be adjusted to meet the needs of communities, especially diverse populations. Research and evaluation activities, in accordance with state and federal laws, professional standards, and institution or organization policies, are one of the main ways health educators contribute to a population's health. Quality education benefits both the health education profession and the general public.

Articles of Code of Ethics in Health Education

Professionals in the health education field are dedicated to promoting excellent healthcare for the individuals, families, groups, organizations, and communities they serve. Improving the human condition and upholding the ethics and integrity of all concerned is the number one priority of health education professionals, along with understanding that all individuals are unique and worth supporting while maintaining their dignity in society.

Health education professionals practice and maintain a code of ethics that is grounded in fundamental principles promoting fairness and integrity and that serves the best interest of people and their families. Health educators must maintain the highest possible standards and encourage ethical behavior with all colleagues regardless of the work setting, professional affiliations, job title, or population served.

Article I: Responsibility to the Public
Educating, promoting, maintaining, and improving the health of individuals, families, groups, and communities is the main responsibility of a health educator. Should a conflict or disagreement arise, the health educator must consider all issues and prioritize those that promote the best health and well-being, while valuing the principles of independence, equality, and human rights for individuals, groups, and communities. Health educators must:
- Support the right of individuals to make informed decisions regarding their health, as long as those decisions do not harm others
- Encourage social practices and actions that support and promote health benefits and eliminate risks for all concerned
- Accurately communicate potential benefits and consequences, if any, associated with the programs and services provided
- Accept responsibility for issues that affect the health of people and their families, groups, and communities
- Be truthful about qualifications, education, expertise, and experience in providing services consistent with his/her professional level and competence
- Respect, ensure, and protect the privacy and dignity of individuals
- Involve people, groups, and communities in the education process to aid understanding and to promote individual responsibility

Article II: Responsibility to the Profession
Promoting ethical conduct and demonstrating professional behavior to maintain the

reputation of the profession is just part of a health educator's job. Health educators must also:

- Improve, maintain, and expand professional knowledge and competence through continued education, participation, and membership in professional organizations related to public health
- Encourage non-discriminatory interactions with others whole maintaining standards of behavior
- Accept responsibility for critical discourse to protect the health education profession
- Refine existing and develop new practices by sharing outcomes of completed work
- Promote transparency of conflicts when both real and perceived conflicts of interest arise
- Appropriately recognize those who contribute information and achieve goals in health education
- Communicate openly to employers, colleagues, and other professionals when they suspect behavior or practices that violate the Code of Ethics

Article III: Responsibility to Employers
Recognizing the boundaries, professional activities, and actions of health educators is only part of a health educator's professional capabilities. He/she must also:

- Accurately represent personal qualifications and those of others in the industry
- Apply guidelines, theories, and current evidence-based standards when performing duties in the field
- Accurately represent program and service outcomes to employers
- Disclose and anticipate conflicts of interest, competing commitments, and product endorsements in the health field
- Openly communicate with employers about job-related assignments and expectations to avoid conflict with professional ethics
- Maintain skills and capabilities in professional practice
- Allocate resources and funds with complete transparency for fiscal responsibility

Article IV: Responsibility in Health Education Delivery
Health education must be delivered with integrity and respect to meet the needs of diverse populations and communities. This delivery includes:

- Being sensitive to cultural and social diversity when planning and implementing programs in the community
- Staying informed of the latest information and advances in health education research and practices
- Using methods and strategies that help develop professional theories, standards, guidelines, experience, and current data
- Evaluating methods and program effectiveness used to achieve results in health education

- Promoting ways to implement a healthful lifestyle through accurate information rather than forcing people to achieve results
- Communicating potential outcomes of proposed strategies, decisions, and services that affect all individuals, groups, and communities
- Communicating and collaborating with other professionals from varied education backgrounds and acknowledging their contributions and skills

Article V: Responsibility in Research and Evaluation

Research and evaluation activities are an ongoing practice that contributes to the health of a population and benefits the health education profession. All research and evaluations must be completed by health educators according to state and federal laws and regulations, organization and institution policies, and professional standards. Health educators must:

- Observe and follow practices and principles when performing evaluations to avoid harming an individual, group, or community including the environment
- Use informed consent to confirm that participation in research is totally voluntary
- Respect the privacy, dignity, and rights of all members involved in the research process and honor commitments to participants
- Keep all participant information confidential and inform participants of disclosure procedures required for research
- Take credit for his/her work, but also recognize the contributions of others
- Evaluate all research objectively, accurately, and timely, so research can be applied where needed
- Share conflicts of evaluation and dissemination in research

Article VI: Responsibility in Professional Preparation

Those involved in training and preparing health educators are obligated to provide quality education that benefits individuals, groups, communities, and the health education profession. Therefore, health educators must:

- Provide equal opportunity for all students and individuals when administering quality education
- Create an educational culture and environment favorable to the health of those involved, free from harassment and discrimination
- Develop and engage in careful planning to present current, accurate, and appropriate material, while providing prompt feedback, stating clear and concise expectations and conducting fair assessments and evaluations
- Provide comprehensive, accurate, and objective counseling to students about career opportunities, while assisting them in securing employment or furthering opportunities for continued education
- Offer adequate supervision and opportunities for learners to continue professional development

Leadership

Leaders in the health education field conduct and sponsor educational programming that offers the most recent and accurate information. Health education leaders are role models and serve as an extension of the professional staff they represent. They must be committed to addressing health issues that are relevant to the community and company they serve. Health issues may include nutrition, sleep and eating disorders, body image, stress, reproductive and sexual health, drugs, tobacco, and/or alcohol abuse.

A health education leader must possess a positive attitude and be able to coordinate a variety of tasks and responsibilities, using appropriate time management skills. A role model for healthy lifestyle choices helps effectively educate everyone about health and wellness issues. A dependable and responsible individual with effective communication skills is necessary in health education, and there will be times when you might have to say, "I don't know the answer to that question, but I will research it and find the answer as soon as possible."

Partnerships

Principles for Creating Effective Partnerships
The essential elements for developing and maintaining a successful, effective partnership are:
1. Mutual trust and respect – establishing a relationship in an effective partnership within an organization and/or community is an ongoing process.
2. Agree on a mission, goals, values, and objectives that serve the organization and community and that yield high quality services in all programs. It is important to realize that changes prioritizing the community over the program may be necessary for best results.
3. Balance power and share resources with all partners involved. Balancing power is the key to a successful, thriving relationship and prevents misunderstandings. This balance may be difficult during times with limited resources and diverse communities and may involve control over grants or real estate issues, for example. Moderating the imbalance of resources and promoting a shift towards attaining common goals helps represent all partners involved.
4. Openly communicate with partners and develop a common language. Recognizing differences at the onset of a partnership and reminding everyone of common goals can help prevent the end of a potentially productive relationship.

Internal and External Resources
Today, state-of-the art health education curriculum reflects essential knowledge needed to shape personal values and beliefs that support healthy behaviors and lifestyles. An effective health education curriculum has the following characteristics:
- **Specific health goals** – including behavioral outcomes directly related to goals

that include instructional strategies and learning experiences for a positive outcome.

- **Theory and research driven** – a positive and effective curriculum extends beyond an intellectual level and addresses social factors, attitudes, norms, values, and skills that influence healthy behaviors.

- **Speaks to individual values, beliefs, and attitudes** –supports positive healthy behaviors and motivates students and learners to examine personal perspectives to generate positive instead of negative perceptions, especially about high-risk behaviors like smoking, for example.

- **Provides instructional strategies** – and learning experiences that help students and learners accurately assess high-risk behaviors, while correcting misperceptions of social norms and emphasizing the value of good health.

- **Reinforces protective factors by increasing perceptions of practicing unhealthy behaviors.** This characteristic allows students and learners to validate positive, healthy intentions and beliefs while understanding the risks of engaging in unhealthy behaviors and situations.

- **Provides opportunity to analyze unhealthy and risky behaviors** that are influenced by media, social barriers, and peer pressures.

- **Builds essential skills** such as communication, planning, goal-setting, assessments of information, accuracy, and self-management that develop confidence and help avoid risky or unhealthy behaviors through feedback and reinforcement. Developing skills that involve real-life situations are rehearsed and practiced for success.

- **Using accurate, credible, and reliable information** to assess risks and clarify attitudes and beliefs, while correcting misconceptions about social norms, helps to identify risky situations and permits relevant discussion to determine the best possible decisions. Essentially, curriculum that provides information for the sole purpose of distributing knowledge will not always change behaviors.

- **Strategies that personalize information** and engage students and learners through interactive sessions like role-playing, problem solving, and group discussions are extremely effective. Personalizing information helps maintain interest and motivation and also addresses diverse learning capabilities and styles. Sharing opinions, thoughts, and feelings helps develop critical thinking skills and encourages creative expression when dealing with health-related concepts.

- **Student needs, concerns, experiences, and current knowledge levels** must be assessed to provide age appropriate information, proper teaching methods, and learning strategies. It must be applicable to a student's daily life and be covered in a logical sequence.

- **Information and activities must include diverse cultures** including race, gender, religion, age, ethnicity, sexual orientation, and physical and mental abilities. Acknowledging cultural diversity is key to highlighting the relevance for students in the community, plus it strengthens intercultural interaction and builds cultural resources for families and communities.

Healthy behavior changes take time, so allocate adequate time for instruction and student learning for a sustained effort that maintains these new actions. Long-lasting results come from learning new skills with reinforcement opportunities for new health-promoting skills; from strategies that build on factors promoting healthy behaviors while engaging families, parents, and peers for positive role models in health-promoting standards; and from assessing and managing health education by teachers who have a personal interest in promoting healthy behaviors and who are comfortable with the content of the curriculum.

Baseline

A lack of baseline data concerning important issues, such as alcohol consumption, smoking, and nutrition, is a central problem for health education. Without important statistics and information, willingness of individuals, groups, and communities to change habits is weak at best. A social survey is one of the best ways to acquire accurate information that will provide a general framework of information to create a collection of baseline data. However, remember that shortcomings of this approach are based on postal zip codes in communities and areas served.

MOU and MOA

MOU stands for Memorandum of Understanding and MOA stands for Memorandum of Agreement. Two parties or partnerships use them for written agreements or a contract; however, many believe an MOA signifies a more meaningful or noteworthy commitment. Both agreements are developed between tribal and municipal governments to benefit a variety of environmental services and to maximize funding available for the community. They both involve finding sources available for each party without duplicating each other's efforts. An MOU/MOA functions as a contract, but is not intended to be an enforceable legal arrangement; however, an MOA can contain legal terms and conditions and can command as much legal authority as a contract.

An MOA is a statement about a specific topic acknowledging cooperation between two or more parties and clarifying each party's roles and responsibilities. Compared to a standard contract, it is an attractive option and is much simpler to use. It helps both parties avoid distrust, potential insult, and possible resentment resulting from asking someone to sign a legal contract. The goal of an MOA is to build a cooperative effort and to establish a partnership based on trust rather than legal obligation. It can be as specific or as general as both parties desire and can lead to a more meaningful goal or relationship. MOAs can help gather funds and services for partnerships so that work can be completed. MOAs do not offer the same protection and assurances as a legal contract, but they do indicate a substantial, sensible obligation for a particular situation.

Process Consultation

Health Education Consultant I
Developing and strengthening skills in application, interpretation, consultation, and planning of programs in health education is an ongoing process. Health education programs, projects, and policies are regularly monitored and evaluated. This position involves:
- Identifying objectives
- Evaluating programs
- Selecting pretesting methods and target groups
- Monitoring program progress and contract compliance
- Coordinating and conducting training programs
- Coordinating inventory of educational resources and materials

Health Education Consultant II
A level II health education consultant provides health education to private and public agencies. The position involves:
- Planning, developing, organizing, monitoring, and evaluating health education programs and projects
- Negotiating contracts with final approval
- Coordinating and conducting training programs
- Leading other education consultants and health-related staff
- Evaluating program standards, policies, and procedures

Health Education Consultant III (Specialist)
This category requires responsibilities in difficult, sensitive, and complex programs and involves recommending policy developments in specific areas of expertise. It requires a highly skilled technical program education and may involve leading professional health staff. Responsibilities may significantly impact local, state, and Federal agencies and may include establishing new programs or modifying existing ones.

This position involves developing, planning, organizing, coordinating, implementing, and evaluating all components of a health education program and of statewide projects. Evaluating and ensuring consistency in statewide programs is essential, as is providing (as a leader) professional and administrative guidance and support to staff.

Health Education Consultant IV (Supervisor)
Supervising a small to large group of health education consultants is just part of this administrative position that includes performing difficult, sensitive, and complex

consultations. Policy and program development work are also a part of this special position.

Laws

Statutes Preventing Discrimination in Employment
Employment laws protect employees from discrimination based on age, race, nationality, gender, sexual orientation, disability, religious, or other reasons. Most employment discrimination laws consist of federal and state statutes; however, there are many other practices that are considered discriminatory and are legally prohibited. They include:
- Transferring, promoting, recalling, and laying off workers
- Compensating, assigning, and classifying employees
- Recruiting workers and posting job openings
- Testing, training, and apprenticeship programs
- Retaliation
- Retirement, pay, and disability leave
- Various types of harassment

The following list includes several federal employment discrimination laws that are well-known and some that are not so well-known. They are:
- The Civil Rights Act of 1964 that prohibits discrimination based on color, gender, national origin, pregnancy, race, religion, and sex, including sexual harassment.
- The Civil Rights Act of 1991 provides for monetary damages in cases of intentional employment discrimination.
- The Age Discrimination in Employment Act (ADEA) protects employees who are 40 years of age or older.
- The Americans with Disabilities Act (ADA) and Rehabilitation Act prohibits discrimination against qualified individuals with disabilities.
- The Equal Pay Act addresses unequal pay related to gender.
- The Family and Medical Leave Act (FMLA) guarantees leave for specific health conditions without jeopardizing the worker's employment.
- Title II of the Genetic Information Nondiscrimination Act (GINA) prohibits discrimination based on genetic information about an applicant, employee, or former employee.

The acts listed above are enforced by the Equal Employment Opportunity Commission (EEOC), which coordinates and supervises all federal equal employment opportunity policies, practices, and regulations. The laws and policies outline procedures required to pursue claims of employment discrimination. A discrimination charge must be filed first with the EEOC or a local Fair Employment Practices Agency (FEPA), if available. Before pursuing a civil lawsuit, an individual must receive, within specific time limits set forth in the policies, a "right to sue" notice from that agency.

Age Discrimination in Employment Act (ADEA)

It is unlawful for an employer to refuse to hire or to discharge anyone with respect to compensation, conditions, terms, or privileges of employment due to age. An employer must not limit, segregate, or classify employees in a way that could deprive an individual of employment opportunities due to age or that could reduce an employee's wage rates. It also forbids discriminating against individuals over the age of forty by refusing to hire them or by making other distinctions based on age. This act covers unions and employment agencies and is enforced by the Equal Employment Opportunity Commission (EEOC).

Americans with Disabilities Act of 1990 (ADA)

The Americans with Disabilities Act forbids discrimination against disabled individuals in employment; local and state government; public accommodations; and commercial facilities, transportation, and telecommunications. To receive ADA protection, a person must have a disability or have a relationship with a disabled individual. The ADA defines a disabled person as someone who has a mental or physical impairment that substantially limits one or more major life activities. The definition also includes a person who is perceived by others as having an impairment or a person who has a history or record of one.

Rehabilitation Act of 1990

Before the ADA, government agencies providing rehabilitative services assumed most people with severe disabilities were not employable; however, now they must assume that such individuals can work. Now, the state rehabilitation program must prove that disabled individuals are not able to work.

Vietnam Veteran's Readjustment Assistance Act of 1974 (VEVRAA)

The Vietnam Veteran's Readjustment Assistance Act (VEVRAA) requires federal government contractors and subcontractors to take affirmative action to employ specified categories of veterans protected by the act, and it prohibits discrimination against such veterans. VEVRAA requires all contractors and subcontractors to list employment openings, and covered veterans receive first priority. An annual report indicating all covered veterans must be submitted. The Employment Standards Administration's Office of Federal Contract Compliance Programs (FCCP) within the U.S. Department of Labor (DOL) enforces affirmative action and mandatory job-listing provisions.

Fair Credit Reporting and Disclosure Act (FCRA)

The federal Fair Credit Reporting Act (FCRA) promotes fairness, accuracy, and privacy of information in consumer reporting agency files. These agencies include credit bureaus and specialty agencies, such as those that sell information about medical records, check-writing histories, and rental history. Here are the main rights under the FCRA:

Everyone must be told if his/her information has been used against them - Any company or individual who uses a credit report or other type of consumer report to deny an application for credit, insurance, or employment must disclose the name, address, and phone number of the agency that provided the information.

Everyone has the right to know what is in his/her file - An individual may request and receive all of his/her information from a consumer-reporting agency file. Of course, proper identification including social security number is required, and many times, this service is free. You are entitled to a free file disclosure if:

- A company or person has taken adverse action against you because of information in your credit report
- You are a victim of identity theft and a fraud alert is placed in your file
- Your file contains inaccurate information because of fraud
- You are unemployed, but expect to apply for employment in the next 60 days
- You are on a public assistance program

All consumers are entitled to a free credit report disclosure every 12 months through each nationwide credit bureau or from a specialty consumer-reporting agency. A consumer-reporting agency may not report negative information that is more than seven years old or bankruptcies that are more than ten years old. They may provide information to an employer, insurer, or creditor when an individual is applying for a job or loan, but only with that individual's written consent.

Immigration Reform and Control Act of 1986
This act was passed to deter and control illegal immigration to the United States. Its major requirement stipulates legalization of aliens who do not have documents, legalization of agricultural workers, increased enforcement of U.S. border crossings, and authorizations for employers who knowingly hire undocumented workers.

Employment Rights
The Department of Labor's Office of Federal Contract Compliance Programs (OFCCP) requires federal contractors and subcontractors to take affirmative action to employ and advance individuals with disabilities. The Americans with Disabilities Act prohibits discrimination by employers against qualified individuals with disabilities. The Equal Employment Opportunity Commission (EEOC) is the primary authority for enforcing employment-related requirements. The Civil Rights Center of the EEOC enforces employment-related requirements and covers organizations that receive federal financial assistance from the Department of Labor. It also enforces workforce-related practices of local and state governments and other public entities.

Family Medical Leave Act 1993 (FMLA)
The Family Medical Leave Act was instated to allow eligible employees to take job-protected leave, with continued group health insurance coverage, for medical or familial reasons. It is unpaid, but entitles employees a leave of absence to give birth to a child; to care for a spouse, parent, or child with a serious health condition; or for a military or serious health condition that makes it impossible to perform a job.

Workers' Compensation

The Department of Labor administers worker's compensation to individuals who are injured at work or who contract a disease from their occupation. It includes wage replacement, medical treatment, vocational rehabilitation, and other benefits. Individuals injured on the job while employed by a private company or local or state government agency should contact their state worker's compensation board for specific information related to their situation. There are several programs designed to prevent work-related injury and illness available through the Department of Labor.

Employee Benefits and Compensation

Employee benefits refer to health, life, and disability insurance; retirement plans; vacation time; and employee stock ownership plans. Benefit options are becoming more limited and are changing because of the business expenses required to provide these benefits. Employee benefits are awarded for completing a job and contributing to a company or organization. Worker's compensation is not necessarily a benefit, but instead is a worker's right. For example, unemployment and worker's compensation are required under federal law. Benefits also include advancement opportunities, a nice office space, and/or appreciation expressed by the boss or owner. Medical insurance is a benefit; however, because of high medical costs, the employee usually pays a part of the cost.

Equal Pay Act of 1963

The Equal Pay Act of 1963 was enacted by Congress to establish a requirement that women be paid equally for equal work. Women's average wages are still lower than men's, and many critics have agreed this act has failed. The idea for the Equal Pay Act began during WWII when many women entered the workforce while men were overseas. The War Labor Board established a policy for equal pay for women that included comparable wages for comparable work; however, it spurred heated debates, and the bill did not pass.

After WWII, Congress reconsidered the issue, and the legislation finally received enough support to be passed into law, amending the Fair Labor Standard Act of 1938. The Equal Pay Act was established by Congress to broaden women's rights. Employers were prohibited from discriminating against women who performed the same jobs as men. The act established that an employer could pay a male employee a higher wage than a female employee if they could establish that payment is based on:

- Seniority
- A merit system
- An earnings system based on the quality and quantity of production by an employee
- A differential based on factors other than employee gender (this factor has been litigated more than the other three in the court system)

Some employers are required to demonstrate a gender-neutral wage policy or a gender-neutral system is enlisted for business reasons. Several courts have noted that the Equal Pay Act does not establish a system of comparable worth because it applies to equal work. The limitations of this act have led to much criticism, but the criticism has highlighted this ongoing issue.

Fair Labor Standards Act (FLSA)
The Fair Labor Standards Act was enacted in 1938 to protect workers by setting standards for minimum wage, overtime pay, record keeping, and youth labor. It covers both full- and part-time workers in the private sector as well as local, state, and federal governments. It is often referred to as enterprise coverage or individual coverage, depending on the type of work you do.

Employee Retirement Income Security Act of 1974 (ERISA)
Enacted in 1974, the Employee Retirement Income Security Act established minimum standards for pension plans in private industries and provided rules on federal income tax effects of transactions associated with benefit plans. The ERISA was formed to protect the interests of employees and their beneficiaries by:
- Requiring the disclosure of financial information concerning beneficiary plans
- Establishing standards of conduct for plan fiduciaries
- Providing appropriate remedies and access to court systems

The responsibilities and enforcement of the ERISA is divided among the Department of the Treasury, the Department of Labor, and the Pension Benefit Guaranty Corporation.

Consolidated Omnibus Budget (COBRA)
Life events can be challenging, especially after losing a job or changing jobs. The Consolidated Omnibus Budget Reconciliation Act (COBRA) was enacted to give workers and their families who lose health benefits the right, under specific circumstances, to continue group health benefits provided by the plan. Generally, COBRA required employer-sponsored group health plans with 20 or more employees to offer the option of temporarily extending health coverage, known as continuation coverage, where the plan would otherwise stop.

It applies to plans sponsored by local and state governments and those in the private sector. The provisions of COBRA are enforced by the Department of Health and Human Services. There are several situations where workers and family members may lose group health coverage, but may be eligible for COBRA coverage. They include:
- Involuntary or voluntary termination of the covered employee for reasons other than gross misconduct
- Work hours are reduced for the covered employee
- The covered employee becomes eligible for Medicare
- Legal separation or divorce of a covered employee
- Dependent child status is lost under the plan

The group health plan benefits under COBRA may be retained for a set period of time, depending on the reason for losing health coverage.

Unemployment Compensation
The Unemployment Compensation Program was created by the Social Security Act of 1935 to provide temporary and partial wage replacements when workers become involuntarily unemployed and to help stabilize economic conditions during recessions. The system is managed by the U.S. Department of Labor, but each state administers its own program. To qualify for benefits, an unemployed person must have worked for a covered employer for a specified time period and have earned a certain amount.

National Labor Relations Act of 1935 (NLRA)
The National Labor Relations Act was passed by Congress to protect the rights of employers and employees, to curtail private sector labor and management practices, to encourage collective bargaining, and to protect the general welfare of businesses and workers in this country.

Findings and Policies

The rights of employees to organize for collective bargaining can lead to strikes and other forms of industrial strife if employers deny those rights. This strife can impair commercial efficiency, safety, and operations; slow the flow of raw materials and manufacturing of goods; affect pricing; and decrease wages and employment. It can aggravate recurrent business slumps by lowering wage rates and purchasing power of wage earners, preventing industry stabilization of competitive wage rates and working conditions.

Protecting the rights of employees to organize and bargain collectively helps prevent injuries and work interruptions and promotes the flow of commerce. Protection by law encourages friendly resolutions to disputes about wages, hours, or other working conditions. It can help restore a balance of bargaining power between employees and employers. United States policy eliminates obstructions to free commercial flow and encourages collective bargaining, while protecting employees.

Worker Adjustment and Retraining Notification Act of 1988 (WARN)
The Worker Adjustment and Retraining Notification Act of 1988 protects workers, families, and communities by requiring employers to give a 60-day notice of closing or mass layoffs within the company. Notice must be given to affected workers, the appropriate local government unit, and the State Dislocated Worker Unit. Employees who work for employers with over 100 workers, not counting those who have worked less than six months in the last year or who work less than twenty hours per week, are covered by WARN. Hourly and salaried workers, as well as management and supervisors, are entitled to notice under WARN; however, business partners are not. The United States district courts enforce the WARN requirements, allowing worker representatives to file individual or class action lawsuits.

The Occupational Safety and Health Act (OSHA) of 1970
The Occupational Safety and Health Administration (OSHA) enforces the Occupational Safety and Health Act (OSH) that covers all employers and employees

in all fifty states, including Puerto Rico and the District of Columbia. Coverage is provided by an OSHA-approved State Job Safety and Health Plan or by the federal Occupational Safety and Health Administration. An employer is any person engaged in a business that affects commerce or is someone who has employees, excluding states and political subdivisions of a state. The act applies to those in:

- Agriculture
- Construction
- Law and medicine
- Manufacturing
- Long shoring
- Charities and disaster relief
- Organized labor
- Private education

The act does not cover self-employed persons, farmers who employ family members, employees of local and state governments, working conditions in nuclear energy, and mining and transportation industries.

HIPAA

The HIPAA Privacy Rule is enforced by the Office for Civil Rights and protects individual privacy and health information. It sets national standards for electronic security systems and for confidentiality stipulations that protect and improve patient safety.

Theories

Strategic Planning in Administering and Managing Health Education

Strategic planning requires a background in and understanding of how the health system works in a health educator's country. The included elements are the health service delivery system, the community, and its operating environment. It requires a systematic process of identifying goals and the appropriate actions to achieve them. Strategic health planning should improve, based on available resources and community needs, the health of a given population and maintain equal and fair health system accessibility.

Successful healthcare organizations are constantly setting and achieving new goals by working with those who can help them expand and identify growth areas. Becoming an industry leader requires cutting-edge services and high-quality staff and health experts. For any given organization, healthcare strategies and recommendations must include feedback, timelines, and objectives. Managing health education in healthcare organizations requires identifying strengths, weaknesses, and growth opportunities and analyzing operations, staffing, and general missions for optimized growth. This includes:

- Service and equipment costs
- Staff recruitment and training
- Marketing and branding

- Labor/training
- Facility maintenance
- Supplies
- Assessments
- Competitive analyses

The analysis of demographic data and market research allows goals to be implemented and supported for optimum growth and stability. Strategic planning and analysis includes summaries of all data and information, healthcare costs, and detailed expense reports. Marketing analysis and planning resources are important parts of strategic planning and health education management, creating a positive presence in a community.

Four Common Critical Questions
What is the National Commission for Health Education Credentialing, Inc. (NCHEC)?
The NCHEC is a non-profit organization whose mission is to enhance the professional practice of health education by promoting and sustaining a credentialed body of health education specialists. The NCHEC certifies health education specialists, promotes professional developments, and strengthens professional preparation and practice. The organization was established in 1988, and today, there are more than 9,000 individuals who are Certified Health Education Specialists (CHES) and Master Certified Health Education Specialists (MCHES).

How can one get involved with the NCHEC?
All active CHES and MCHES candidates are eligible to seek nomination each spring for positions on the Board of Commissioners and other Division Boards. More information and available opportunities are available on the NCHEC website. For specific committee functions and availabilities, contact the executive director.

What is a Certified Health Education Specialist (CHES)?
A Certified Health Education Specialist is an individual who has met all eligibility requirements and has successfully passed a competency-based examination demonstrating knowledge and skill of 7 areas of responsibility. The 7 areas of responsibility are:
  Area I: Assess Needs, Assets, and Capacity for Health Education
  Area II: Plan Health Education
  Area III: Implement Health Education
  Area IV: Conduct Evaluation and Research Related to Health Education
  Area V: Administer and Manage Health Education
  Area VI: Serve as a Health Education Resource Person
  Area VII: Communicate and Advocate for Health and Health Education

What is a Master Certified Health Education Specialist (MCHES)?
A Master Certified Health Education Specialist is an individual who has met all academic eligibility requirements through courses in health education and experience

in the health education field. He/she has passed a comprehensive written examination and is committed to professional development and advanced-level continuing education.

Ten Steps

Step 1: Gain Support from Management

Management support is critical for ensuring a health education program is backed by an organization and has suitable human and financial resources available. Success depends on support from leaders, including managers, who embrace the program, and employees follow suit. Committees or groups are formed as part of a health education program. Gaining support depends on building a strong business case for the program including:

- How a health education program would benefit the organization
- Improved employee health through physical activity and good nutrition
- Costs to an organization when poor nutrition and lack of exercise are related to employee absenteeism and poor performance
- Knowing the resources required to organize and support the program effectively
- Anticipating results and overall outcomes
- Using examples of successful programs in other organizations

Step 2: Introduce the Concept and Identify Specific Needs

To ensure program success, all employees must be engaged. If it is relevant to specific employee needs, it will help a health education specialist understand an organization's work environment. Identify priorities and develop a program to meet employee goals and objectives. This will help evaluate the program's success. You can use focus groups to identify employee issues, preferences, and ideas or to take a health and wellness survey of the workplace environment. When assessing needs and concerns, employees who work remotely should also be considered and included.

Step 3: Gain Support From Employees and Establish Program Responsibilities

Employees need to understand the benefits of a health education program, which may require you to outline the benefits for both the organization and its employees. This involves identifying who is responsible for coordinating a program and who is willing to promote the program to their colleagues. If the organization is large, establishing a committee or working group may be necessary to coordinate program development, which is a great way to generate ideas and share responsibilities while keeping it manageable.

Step 4: Develop Goals and Objectives

Identifying and clearly stating program goals will help focus on the needs and interests of the organization and its employees. It will help with expected outcomes and with resources (time and money) required to achieve these outcomes.

Step 5: Identify Program Activities and Develop an Action Plan with a Budget

Activities should address the primary interests and needs of employees while maintaining a budget and timeline for your program. Activities can be very simple and inexpensive like organizing a walking group at lunchtime or a yoga class where everyone brings his/her own mat. Some activities may require more time and resources to implement, such as weight-bearing exercises or other specialty classes. Including a range of activities is important to increase participation and meet employee needs.

Step 6: Select Rewards and Incentives for Program Participation

Rewards and incentives can motivate and increase participation in a health education program, providing a reason for changing behaviors and improving program loyalty. The following items are ideas for rewards and incentives:

- Certificates and prizes for those who make the effort to change and who participate regularly
- Competitions for each day of participation or for weight lost
- Acknowledging those at meetings or events who have achieved success in an activity
- Providing healthy merchandise like water bottles, towels, and gift certificates to local businesses, that will enhance program efforts
- Cash incentives to increase participation
- Launching an activity or event during lunch or morning tea to initiate events
- Offering time off at work for participating
- Using a point system to redeem incentives or vouchers
- Providing gift certificates for dinner as a reward

Step 7: Identify Additional Support to Implement Program

Support from other resources, such as your local health department or state or national agencies, can help implement a program in your organization. They include:

- Fact sheets and brochures to use as tools
- Sporting clubs and local gyms
- Physical activity programs, such as walk-a-thons, that involve the entire community
- American Heart Association's Guide to Healthful Eating

Step 8: Promote Your Program to Employees

Promoting your program will raise awareness and generate interest for participation by advertising activities and events. It will help motivate employees to participate and will increase motivation for long-term success. Promoting the program or event inspires employees, especially if management is supportive and the program is launched using a guest speaker, local expert, nutritionist, or health coach. Newsletters are an effective way to provide information and promote activities and events through employee emails. Create a place online where employees can share their program experiences.

Step 9: Manage Your Program by Enacting Your Plan

Once all developmental steps have been completed for your program, it is time to enact your plan by holding regular meetings, coordinating and arranging for event and activity support, managing the budget, and continuing to promote each event through email and newsletters.

Step 10: Evaluate Each Program

Evaluating each program allows you to review their effectiveness and to make any needed improvements. It will help determine if goals and objectives are being achieved. Ask employees questions to determine what they like and don't like about a particular event or activity. You might ask:
- Was the event or activity delivered as planned?
- What changes or improvements would you like to see?
- What was the effect of the program?
- What activities were most popular?

Evaluating each program and activity is essential to discovering what employees do and don't like, which will help continue to improve the program. Knowing what does and doesn't work is key to making the right decisions for the future of the employees and the program.

Generalized Model for Program Planning

Understanding and Engaging
⇓
Assessing Needs
⇓
Setting Goals and Objectives
⇓
Developing an Intervention
⇓
Implementing the Intervention
⇓
Evaluating the Results

Cost Analysis is a technique used to evaluate the economics of a program and involves collecting, categorizing, and analyzing the program's costs including costs of illness.

Cost-Effectiveness Analysis is an evaluation method used when only one program is being assessed or if information about the program's effectiveness is unavailable. The interventions being assessed and compared are equally effective and allow researchers to minimize costs for the programs under consideration. The goal is to identify the least expensive method to achieve goals and objectives.

Cost-Benefit Analysis is the value of all resources including supplies, labor, equipment, and buildings used to produce a product or service. The true program cost is not only the total expenses, but also the value of the benefits that would have been provided if the resources were used for other purposes.

Quality versus Cost
Quality health education is important and does cost money; however, people cannot avoid either expense. The government is involved in healthcare and education because a real market would possibly reject people and employees without providing the medical care or education they need. The government subsidizes healthcare and education because of high costs. The quality of a health education program outweighs the monetary costs because it can reduce long-term healthcare costs. The more options people have for maintaining their health, the less expensive healthcare will be for everyone.

Budgets
Supporting budgets are a way of enabling an organization to become involved with how resources are used, allocated, and spent when addressing the needs of employees and staff. Advocating health budgets is about campaigning to change the way resources are used to deliver health education. Health budget advocacy can help you identify failures and inequities among different populations and levels of care. Involving a broad group of individuals or stakeholders in decision-making, especially those affected directly, can lead to successful outcomes.

Examples of Budget Reports
A budget should accurately reflect the costs of any proposed education, service, or research program. It provides the sponsoring agency information about why costs are necessary and about how they are met. Financial data is analyzed to determine which costs are allocated to which program, allowed under federal guidelines and treated consistently by the organization or institution.

For example, when a university receives an award, an agreement is made between the sponsor and the university. Only those costs included in the budget and allowed by the sponsor should be directly charged to the award and shown in the budget. If a cost requires approval, it must be secured before any costs are incurred. It is important to develop a budget that supports all program requirements.

A budget must support:
- Proposed direct costs
- Proposed cost share
- Estimated program income including projected revenue and expenditures
- Facilities and administration (F&A or indirect costs)

Funding Sources
When developing a budget, the first step is to determine a funding source, whether it flows through state or local governments or through the private sector. The College of Public Health (COPH) Department of Research can help grant writers identify funding sources.

Federal/Federal Flow-Through
If funding comes from a federal source, the budget must comply with sponsoring agency guidelines, OMB Circular A-21, and Cost Principles for Educational Institutions. Costs, including direct costs related to any production, must be determined so that all resources can be reasonably allocated.

Non-Federal Sources
Budgets developed for non-federal funding sources must comply with sponsor agency budget guidelines and university guidelines.

A Sample Budget Justification
A budget must adhere to guidelines provided by the sponsoring agency and is intended to help principal investors, investigators, and project personnel develop budget explanations that will enable reviewers to thoroughly analyze budget requests according to program criteria. The following areas are usually included:
- Facilities and administration or indirect costs
- Salaries and wages
- Contractual costs
- Fringe benefits
- Consultant costs
- Equipment
- Supplies
- Travel
- Other (to be defined)

Grants
Grants improve healthcare access by helping health profession training programs address pressing needs among workers and employees. Healthcare programs encourage distribution to under-served areas, increase diversity among racial and ethnic minorities, and develop programs that meet the needs of all groups including young and old individuals and those with disabilities. Most grants in the health profession go to universities and colleges to build programs to enroll diverse students. Each program has specific eligibility requirements; however, private and public hospitals, non-profit organizations, and health profession schools are eligible to apply.

Elements of a Grant Proposal
A grant proposal must convince the prospective donor that a significant problem exists and that the specific agency can meet the need and/or solve the problem. The proposal should be no longer than 15 pages and should include the following:
- Qualifications of the specific organization
- Needs assessment or statement of the problem
- Goals and objectives of the program
- Method for achieving goals
- Evaluation of the program
- Funding for the future

- Budget

Letter of Intent or Inquiry

Some organizations, corporations, or foundations prefer a letter of inquiry to determine whether the applicant is eligible. The letter should be concise and without attachments. If the organization determines the project is appropriate, it will direct the grant writer to submit a complete proposal. If not, a refusal letter will be issued at that time. A letter of inquiry should include the following:

- A name, title, address, and phone number
- Be addressed to the individual responsible for the funding
- A brief overview of the organization and its purpose
- The reason for the funding request and the amount
- A description of the needs to be met by the project, including target population and statistics
- A brief project description
- A list of other prospective funders for the project
- Thank the individual and offer the next step to be taken
- All contact information
- A signature

Full Proposal Cover Letter

The cover letter serves as an introduction to the organization and should always accompany a proposal. A cover letter should include the following:

- The funder's name, title, and address
- A brief overview of the organization and its purpose
- The reason for the funding request, including the amount
- Be one page only
- The organization's name, address, and phone number
- Letter writer's signature

The Summary

This part of the proposal should concisely summarize the request to help the reader visualize the project. The remainder of the proposal will deepen the understanding of the vision presented in the summary. It should appear at the beginning of the proposal and should identify the grant applicant. Include at least one sentence about each of the following:

- Credibility
- The problem
- Objectives
- Methods
- Total cost

Write clearly, concisely and make it interesting, but limit it to half a page. The qualifications for funding establish credibility, highlighting accomplishments of the organization's programs including how specific issues were handled and addressed.

Clearly state why the organization requesting funds should conduct the project and how it is capable of solving the problem or meeting the needs of the organization. A proposal should be based on the need for the project and on methodology, not the accomplishments of the organization.

If growth is expected over the next year, then anticipated goals should be stated including an annual report, if it exists. The qualifications of the organization should include the following:

- Who is applying for funding
- The rationale for the organization's founding
- The agency's purpose and long-term goals
- Current programs and activities
- Clients
- Applicant's accomplishments (including support or documentation)
- Endorsements of accomplishments
- Qualifications of key staff members
- Problem statement
- Be brief and interesting

Needs Assessment or Problem Statement

A specific problem or need must be addressed and researched information must be provided to justify the problem or need. The provided data should be convincing, but not too overwhelming or lengthy. A needs assessment or problem statement should include the following:

- The target population to be served
- The need or problem addressed
- Goals and purpose of the applicant's agency or organization
- Relevant evidence
- Needs and problems stated in the client's terms, not the applicant's
- Be brief and to the point
- Make a compelling case

Organizations

Mission Statements

Mission statements must clearly state what an organization or unit is trying to achieve. A mission statement also should reflect the difference you want to make. Concrete goals will motivate and inspire those involved in the organization.

Organizational Support

Organizational support refers to employees' perception concerning their performance and well-being and to the value of their contribution to an organization's goals and work.

Organizational Culture

The organization's expectations, experiences, philosophy, and values are expressed in its image, inner-workings, and interactions with the outside world. All of these are based on shared beliefs, attitudes, customs, and rules that have been developed over time and are considered an integral part of an organization. The culture of an organization is always unique and one of the hardest parts to change.

Five Aspects

The five aspects of an organization include the following:
1. The way the organization conducts business and treats customers and employees.
2. How often new ideas are welcome, decision-making, and personal expression.
3. How information and power flow through the hierarchy of the organization.
4. How dedicated and committed employees are towards common goals and objectives.
5. How performance and productivity affect the organization, from client care and service to product quality and safety.

Capacity for Change

Capacity for change can be defined as the organization's total amount of work for operating daily and changing those activities. Adding new work requirements or duties can affect daily operations in several ways. If demands extend beyond people's capabilities or capacities, your best talent may become stressed, resentful, and may depart, or those employees may display poor performance and increasing failures from lack of time. Most organizations reward operational performance rather than change the system.

Capacity for change becomes an issue when normal operations are strained and more work continues to be added. Additionally, mandating major changes requiring resources, meetings, personal changes, and planning on top of normal operating procedures can dramatically affect an organization.

Organizational Climate

Properties of an organization observed by employees strongly influence their actions and job performance. A good leader might survey employees to identify and promote aspects that are most important in achieving the organization's goals.

Organizational Capacity

The capacity of an organization describes the wide range of knowledge, capabilities, and resources needed to effectively achieve goals and objectives.

Layers within an Organization

The majority of companies and organizations start out lean; however, over time, they find that complexity creeps in through layers that accumulate. The distance between leadership and the frontline can increase and lead to higher costs. Moreover, ideas and decisions tend to stop flowing as smoothly throughout the organization. Even some of the best-performing organizations discover that, to be more effective, they must reduce layers.

Subsystems
Subsystems are the life functions necessary for the organization to exist in a changing environment.

Diffusion of Innovations
Diffusion is the process by which an innovative idea or plan is communicated through certain channels within an organization. Each person involved in the decision-making process bases that decision on knowledge, implementation, and confirmation of a plan or objective.

Human Resources and Health Education Standards (HES)
Unifying core values of safety, integrity, and respect for people and the environment are an integral part of administering and managing health education. Specific responsibilities are assigned to directors, leaders, and employees to fulfill this commitment. A formal health, environment, and safety management system provides the means and resources to manage HES programs. It encourages individual responsibility, values quantifiable results, and promotes communication with employees and others involved in the program.

Human Resources for which HES may be responsible include:
- Complying with laws and regulations
- Enhancing employee safety performance
- Minimizing environmental effects and risks
- Meeting objectives and sustaining improved performance

Internal versus External Assessments
An internal assessment is often called a "teacher-made test" or "home examination." The aim of an internal assessment is to evaluate student or employee progress in different programs at different levels. Educators frame the exam questions, complete the exam, and examine the answers. The objectives of an internal assessment are to:
- Evaluate learned concepts
- Estimate progress and the ability to learn
- Promote those concepts within, based on an internal exam
- Foster a competing environment that creates a positive effect
- Evaluate curriculum
- Study further in a particular area, if needed
- Develop hidden abilities, capabilities, desires, and interests for guidance

A type of internal assessment might be a weekly, monthly, or annual exam that can be related to the work being completed. An internal assessment allows feedback, identifies areas needing improvement in those involved, and is helpful with decisions regarding promotion.

External Assessment

An external assessment is organized and conducted by an external agency through standardized tests, observation, and other techniques. The process of an external assessment involves choosing the questions, paper, and examination centers and distributing exams. It allows for on-the-spot evaluation where head examiners mark the exam for completion. The importance and objectives of an external assessment include:

- A degree or certificate
- Comparing abilities
- Evaluating an institution's progress
- Attaining employment for selection of intelligent educators and employees
- Competing
- Evaluating objectives and curriculum
- Creating good habits in employees

Stages of Team Development and Leadership Actions

Forming

The FIRST STAGE of team developing involves forming a team that meets and learns about the opportunities and challenges, agrees on goals, and begins to tackle the assigned tasks. During the first stage, team members are usually on their best behavior and are often focused on themselves. Team leaders must direct and guide so that objectives and goals are clear to all involved. The first stage is also the time when everyone gets to know each other and how team members interact and respond to direction.

Storming

The STORMING STAGE comes next and is where different ideas compete for consideration. The team addresses issues and problems that need to be solved. Team members also determine how they will function both independently and together. Team member ideas and perspectives are confronted and in some cases, the storming stage is resolved quickly, depending on the maturity level of team members. The team must grow through this stage to resolve their differences and to participate more comfortably. As everyone shares his/her particular opinions and views, struggle, tension, and sometimes heated arguments can occur.

Norming

The NORMING STAGE is when the team manages to arrive at a mutual agreement and plan for the team. Some team members must forget their own ideas and agree with others to help the team function and achieve goals and objectives. In this stage, individual responsibility ensures that the team achieves its goals.

Performing

The PERFORMING STAGE is when a team is able to function as a unit and can find ways to complete the job effectively and smoothly without conflict or the need for supervision. The team is knowledgeable and motivated, with competent team members working together and making decisions without supervision. Typically, supervisors are still involved on a participative level; however, the team will make most of the required decisions. Commonly, teams revert back to the earlier stages and sometimes enter cycles when reacting to changes in circumstances. For example, this situation can occur after a change in leadership when team members are compelled to challenge existing team dynamics and norms.

Organizational Development Theory (ODT)

The Organizational Development Theory is a field of theory, research, and practice dedicated to expanding the effective knowledge of people to achieve higher levels of performance and change in an organization. ODT is a process of ongoing action planning, diagnosis, implementation, and evaluation and has a main goal of transferring knowledge and skills to health education organizations to improve problem solving and manage future changes.

Stage Theory

Students must progress through developmental stages in critical thinking to improve thinking and make smart decisions. When properly cultivated through predictable stages, the quality of student work will improve. Passing through these stages is important for developing new levels of intellectual thought that lead to success.

Inter-Organizational Relations Theory

Inter-Organizational Relations theory relates to the efforts to study different aspects of learning and offers a better understanding of how to manage those aspects. Part of the challenge is that they appear in different forms including joint ventures, alliances, trade associations, and networks. However, they do provide a valuable framework from which research can build a positive future.

Networks

A network is a collection of people who are connected to each other through some sort of relationship. Many organizations can be part of a network that consists of people, projects, documents, and organizations. All of these different entities can be linked through a transmission of information, goods, influence, and more. Examples of networks can be seen in development projects, staff, activities, workshops, training events, and email newsletters. People in a network are linked by common concerns and specific objectives.

Model of Network Development

A model of network development clearly identifies who is involved at each level of a project. It identifies how each individual is expected to interact with others, making it easier to understand the overall goals and objectives. Identifying each person makes it possible to develop a network model for each project.

Employee Relations

Employee relations involve maintaining employer-employee relationships that contribute to acceptable productivity, motivation, and morale of all involved. The main aim of employee relations is to prevent problems and solve issues that may affect work conditions.

Recruitment

Recruitment is the process of attracting, screening, selecting, and hiring qualified individuals who meet an organization's needs. Stages of the recruitment process include:

- Analyzing the job
- Sourcing candidates who meet job requirements
- Screening individuals through testing skills
- Assessing a candidate's motivation and how he/she will fit into the organization
- Making and finalizing job offers

Evaluation of Qualifications

Evaluating qualifications occurs during the interview process where appropriate questions and issues are addressed to evaluate prospective health education professionals. Here is a list of questions to consider for this process. They include:

- What type of education/training does the candidate have?
- Note graduation date, all degrees, and type of specialty certification
- Titles of continuing education courses completed in the last two years
- Where and when licensed, registered, or certified (ask for documentation)
- Years of experience in occupational health
- In what industries has the candidate gained experience?
- What management experience(s) has the candidate had? For how long?
- What does the candidate know about OSHA record-keeping requirements?
- Has the candidate ever prepared for and/or participated in an OSHA inspection?
- Does the candidate know about workers' compensation laws in your state?
- Is the candidate familiar with the Americans with Disabilities Act?
- What kind of information does the candidate want to know about your business?
- How can the candidate develop or improve your safety and health program?

Phases of Recruitment

Step 1: Assessing the Need

Determining the need of employees or staffing in an organization is the first step in the recruitment process. Rapid growth might be a future possibility or currently, without enough people to provide the required services, the staff is overworked. Defining your service area or expertise also helps assess need.

Step 2: Use Health Professional Shortage Area Information

The Health Resources and Services Administration Bureau of Health Professions' National Center for Health Workforce Analysis develops criteria and uses it for specific populations and groups.

Step 3: Gain Support
It is important to gain support for recruitment efforts from leaders in your industry or health education field.

Step 4: Form Recruitment Team
It may be necessary to create a recruitment team that gets involved in the recruitment process, which can be a part of success.

Step 5: Define Opportunity
Defining your opportunity will help you define and understand the strengths and weaknesses of your offer compared to the competition. It will also help you identify the right candidates for each position.

Step 6: Define Benefits
A compensation plan is essential for continued growth and success and includes any position benefits, whether medical or other fringe benefits. Financial and professional incentives should be considered and evaluated.

Step 7: Define Your Candidate
Who is your ideal candidate? What professional qualifications or personal traits should this person possess? A brainstorming session may be required to gather key team members to select the right person.

Step 8: Create a Recruitment Budget
A budget will show the costs required, if any, to recruit the right candidate for the job. It may involve advertising in specific places to recruit the perfect candidate.

Step 9: Recruiting the Candidates
Schedule time slots for each interview and determine if there will be an elimination round for each applicant.

Step 10: Screening Candidates
Screening the candidates includes interviewing each candidate and checking his/her references and credentials. The initial screening step is usually completed during the first telephone call. During that call, determine if a candidate is interested in the position and if he/she is qualified and/or suitable for the position.

Training
Training and educational programs will help broaden employee knowledge with educational materials that will enhance employee work and organization goals and objectives. Training courses, educational programs, and training materials should be an ongoing process.

On-the-job training involves learning information that will enhance work, creating a knowledgeable staff and employees who are empowered by what they learn. Off-the-job training involves certifications and training programs outside of the workplace that will enhance work performance and experience.

Conflict Resolution

Conflict resolution is the processes and methods used to facilitate a peaceful, satisfactory ending to a conflict. Many times, members of a group will convey their intentions and reasons for certain beliefs; however, resolving a conflict may require negotiations, mediation, arbitration, and intervention to peacefully resolve a conflict. Conflict and dispute resolution are terms, often used interchangeably, that encompass non-violent measures to promote an effective resolution.

Team-Building Activities

Team-building activities help improve communication between members by helping them understand each other, can boost morale, and are effective learning tools to improve productivity and performance. Learning each other's strengths and weaknesses promotes better teamwork for greater success. Team-building activities include:

- Problem solving
- Decision-making activities
- Building trust
- Communication

An example of a team-building activity is called the Life Highlights Game. First, ask each person to close his/her eyes for one minute and consider the best moment of his/her life. It could be a moment alone or with family or friends, or be professional success, or be an adventure experienced on a trip. Next, ask each participant to take thirty seconds to decide which moment he/she would like to relive if he/she had only 30 seconds left to live. Then, the leader of this activity asks each person what his/her 30 seconds entailed and why he/she chose it. This single activity allows participants to understand each other's personalities and passions.

Community Empowerment and Organizing

Working with Volunteers

Working with volunteers offers a unique opportunity to meet other people in the community and can lead to contacts in business and health education. You might use digital communication to communicate or, if you are located in a rural community, word-of-mouth can be effective. Consider the types of volunteers you would like to work with (this may depend on the specific project in mind).

Recruitment Ideas

- Post online: Volunteermatch.org, local newspapers, community calendars, social media (Facebook, Twitter, Google +, etc.)
- Post fliers around the project area
- Ask friends, family, and co-workers
- Present to local civic groups such as Rotary, Garden Club, etc.

- Ask local businesses to participate
- Contact local schools
- Contact faith-based groups

Four Key Tasks When Working with Volunteers
Working with volunteers can be challenging; however, if used properly, it can provide tremendous advantages.

- **Volunteers save money** – depending on the project or event, volunteer labor can complete a lot of work without charging much money.
- **Volunteers bring needed skills** – such as computer knowledge, organization, or special occasion skills or mediation services that might be needed occasionally.
- **Volunteers bring renewed energy and excitement to an event or project** – that can help revitalize your staff members and rejuvenate the group.
- **Volunteers increase community ownership** – support of your work can be found in the community and can relate to what the community wants or needs.

Volunteering brings together people from different cultures. Health education decisions that affect diverse cultures, ages, and geographic areas of the country can sometimes create conflicts. Each of us uses our values to help guide our decisions. Research of successful volunteers has identified an essential set of core personality traits: flexibility or adaptability, patience, openness, innovativeness, and integrity.

Ecological Approaches to Behavior Change
- The socio-ecological model recognizes the interwoven relationship between an individual and his/her environment.
- While individuals are responsible for instituting and maintaining the lifestyle changes necessary to reduce risk and improve health, individual behavior is determined, to a large extent, by social environment (e.g. community norms and values, regulations, and policies).
- Barriers to healthy behaviors are shared among a community as a whole. As these barriers are lowered or removed, behavior change becomes more achievable and sustainable. It becomes easier to "push the ball up the hill."
- The most effective approach leading to healthy behaviors is a combination of efforts at all levels: individual, interpersonal, organizational, community, and public policy.

Organizational Development
Organizational development is a well-planned effort to increase an organization's efficiencies and effectiveness. It is about promoting organizational readiness to meet the challenges of the future or to effect change through systematic learning and developing strategies that help with beliefs and attitudes. The structure of an organization must be able to absorb new technologies that will help with change. The main purpose of organizational development is to develop the organization through systems and structures, not to conduct training or personal or staff development.

Chapter 6: Serve as a Health Education Resource Person

Introduction

A health education resource person educates people about health and includes both individuals and groups of people promoting, maintaining, and restoring good health. The profession involves the following areas of health:

- Environmental
- Physical
- Social
- Emotional
- Spiritual
- Intellectual

It is a combination of planned learning experiences based on sound science and theories that provide individuals, groups, and communities the opportunity to learn information and skills required to make sound health decisions. This involves some sort of communication designed to improve health literacy, knowledge, and skills conducive to good health for individuals, groups, and communities.

Code of Ethics

The health education profession is dedicated to excellence in the practice of promoting individual, family, organizational, and community health. The Code of Ethics provides a framework of shared values within which health education is practiced. The responsibility of each health educator is to aspire to the highest possible standards of conduct and to encourage the ethical behavior of all his/her colleagues.

Article I: Responsibility to the Public A health educator's ultimate responsibility is to educate people for the purpose of promoting, maintaining, and improving individual, family, and community health. When a conflict arises among individuals, groups, organizations, agencies, or institutions, health educators must consider all issues and prioritize those that promote wellness and living quality through principles of self-determination and freedom of choice for the individual.

Article II: Responsibility to the Profession Health educators are responsible for their professional behavior, for the reputation of their profession, and for promoting ethical conduct among their colleagues.

Article III: Responsibility to Employers Health educators recognize the boundaries of their professional competence and are accountable for their professional activities and actions.

Article IV: Responsibility in the Delivery of Health Education Health educators promote integrity in the delivery of health education. They respect the rights, dignity, confidentiality, and worth of all people by adapting strategies and methods to the needs of diverse populations and communities.

Article V: Responsibility in Research and Evaluation Health educators contribute to the health of the population and to the profession through research and evaluation activities. When planning and conducting research or evaluation, health educators do so according to federal and state laws and regulations, organizational and institutional policies, and professional standards.

Article VI: Responsibility in Professional Preparation Those involved in preparing and training health educators have an obligation to accord learners the same respect and treatment given other groups by providing quality education that benefits the profession and the public.

Fundamental ethical principles to be followed are:
1. Principally, public health should address the fundamental causes of disease and the requirements for health with the goal of preventing adverse health outcomes.
2. Individual rights should always be respected in the community, with regards to public health.
3. Policies, programs, and priorities should be developed and evaluated through health education processes that ensure an opportunity for input from community members.
4. Public health should advocate and work to empower disenfranchised community members with the goal of ensuring that basic resources and conditions necessary for health are accessible to all.
5. Public health should seek information needed to implement effective policies and programs that protect and promote health education.
6. Public health institutions should provide communities with needed information for decisions on policies or programs and should obtain the community's consent for their implementation.
7. Public health education institutions should act in a timely manner on information within their resources and the mandate given by the public.
8. Public health education programs and policies should incorporate a variety of approaches that anticipate and respect diverse values, beliefs, and cultures in the community.
9. Public health education programs and policies should be implemented in a manner that most enhances the physical and social environment.
10. Public health education institutions should protect the confidentiality of information that can harm an individual or community if publicized. Exceptions must be justified based on a high likelihood of significant harm to an individual or others.
11. Public health education institutions should ensure the professional competence of their employees and staff members.

12. Public health education institutions and their employees should engage in collaborations and affiliations in ways that build the public's trust and the institution's effectiveness.

Learning

Learning is obtaining and developing new or reinforcing existing knowledge, skills, behaviors, preferences, and values that may involve fusing or creating different types of information. Learning is contextual, not compulsory and does not happen all at once. It is built on what we already know and may be viewed as a process, rather than collecting facts or procedural knowledge.

Partnering and its Benefits

Partnering with other organizations throughout a community allows opportunities to share knowledge, expertise, talent, equipment, and buildings that benefit all involved. It creates a cohesive situation between health educators and individuals and groups served, benefitting members in the community. Partnering gives access to a full spectrum of resources and services through programs, activities, and professional resources that can benefit those involved. A powerful network can be formed through partnering with others who share the same goals of achieving optimum health through education, grants, scholarships, awards, and other special programs. Diversified personal benefits including financial programs and group discounts add to the benefits of partnering.

Voluntary Health Organization

Voluntary health organization is involved in health education draw from the environmental, psychological, biological, physical, and medical sciences to promote health and prevent disease, disability, and premature death. These organizations accomplish this by educating individuals, groups, and communities to change behaviors to improve well-being and health. The purpose of a voluntary health organization is to positively influence health behaviors and the living conditions and work environments that influence health.

In voluntary health organizations, by focusing on prevention, health education can reduce costs, both human and financial, that individuals, employers, companies, medical facilities, communities, the state, and the nation might spend on medical treatment. A health educator can work in schools, in hospitals or clinics, with community organizations, with non-profit agencies, with companies, or with governmental agencies. Health educators work to promote better overall health on individual, community, and policy levels.

Foundation

A foundation, including those of charities, is a legal classification or category of non-profit organizations that usually donate funds and support other organizations through charitable means. A non-profit organization is different from a private foundation (which is typically endowed by a family or an individual).

DEBI
This stands for Diffusion of Effective Behavioral Interventions. It is intended to provide high-quality training and on-going technical assistance for various health prevention programs throughout communities. It can be accomplished through both intervention and control groups to achieve positive outcomes. Researchers provide input and materials necessary to implement interventions with appropriate training and service providers to achieve effectiveness in prevention programs in communities.

RTIPs
Determining what to do about health, travel, and dental benefits is one of the most important decisions you will make in retirement. There are a lot of factors to consider, and it is sometimes difficult knowing where to begin. RTIP offers five plans, each with a different prescription drug maximum, which all include extended healthcare protection including travel and the option to add dental coverage at any time.

There are many plans available, so begin by determining your current annual prescription drug costs. If you aren't sure, call your pharmacist; he/she can help. Once you have this number, you will be able to review several plan options and choose the plan that best suits you and your family.

SAMHSA
This stands for Substance Abuse and Mental Health Services Administration. They coordinate efforts to reduce behavioral health disparities for diverse populations by creating strategies and data to improve health including grant-making operations and policy development. The goal is to have high-quality behavioral healthcare equally available for all populations and to reduce the impact of substance abuse and mental illness so individuals and families can thrive in a healthy community.

Provide Training

Requests for Training – What should a CHES do upon receiving a request for training?
Identifying needs, assets, goals, and resources of an organization or group is important after receiving a request for training. Assessing resources and needs should be done regularly to serve a specific group or population. The best way to assess needs and assets is by using as many of the available sources of information as possible. It depends on how easily information is found and collected and how much your resources--mostly of people, money, and time--will support. Developing a plan will allow you to consider these obstacles and use the results to determine goals, devise methods, and create a structure for a community assessment that will give you information needed to conduct a successful effort. The following guidelines, while presented in a step-by-step order, may end up in a different sequence, or you may find yourself carrying out two or more steps at once or switching the order of some steps.

1. **Recruit a Planning Group That Represents All Stakeholders and Reflects the Diversity of the Community**. Try to find a true representation of the group or

community that needs to be assessed. This may include low-income people or immigrants that you actually want to participate, especially if they've been cheated by insincere offers in the past. It's worth your time and effort to understand all aspects of the community. Community members are more apt to trust that process and support its results if they are part of the process.

This is also the time to think about whether the planning group will oversee the assessment. That arrangement often makes the most sense, but not always. If the planning group won't be the coordinating body, then part of its planning process should determine the individuals who will be in that group and how to assemble it.

Another important determination at this point is whether the planning group and those who will conduct the assessment (including activities such as contacting informers, constructing surveys, facilitating meetings, gathering data, and reporting on and evaluating the assessment process) will need training, and if so, how much and of what kind.

Many people without much formal education belong to groups that are often denied a voice in community affairs or belong to a culture outside the mainstream and don't have the meeting and deliberation skills that several middle-class citizens do. They might need training and/or mentoring to learn how to contribute effectively to a planning group. Additionally, several people may need training in data collection methods, evaluation, and other areas important to the assessment process. All required training must be anticipated and arranged so that it is completed in a timely and useful manner. Now is the time to start thinking about it.

2. **Design an Evaluation Process for the Assessment, Including the Development of the Plan**. Evaluation should start at the beginning of an effort so that plans can be adjusted and monitored for any possible improvements, ensuring that all work is effective.

3. **Decide WHY You Want to Conduct the Assessment**. There are a number of reasons a community assessment of needs and resources must be done. These include:
- Determining how to address the needs of a particular group or individual.
- Conducting a community health assessment to launch a public health campaign or combat a particular disease or condition.
- Exploring how to affect the activities of a coalition of service providers or government agencies.
- Understanding community needs and resources as a guide to advocacy efforts or policy change. You can't make credible policy recommendations without knowing about current conditions and the current policies affecting them.
- Assessing the impact, intensity, and distribution of a particular issue to create strategies for approaching it. This process may involve breaking down the issue still further and investigating only a part of it, rather than looking at the entire health issue.

- The reasons for an assessment will affect from whom and how you gather information, what is assessed, and what you do with that information. It's important to start planning with a clear understanding of what you want to do so that your plan matches your goals.

4. Determine What Data is Already Available. There is probably a good deal of pre-existing information about a particular group or community. Here are some resources to consider:
- National Institutes of Health
- Centers for Disease Control
- Department of Health and Human Services
- U.S. Census Bureau
- County health rankings for each county
- Local government agencies
- Chamber of Commerce
- Hospitals and Human Service Providers
- Charitable organizations
- Local universities and colleges

It's important that to ensure that whatever data exists is timely. If it's more than six months to a year old, it's out of date and no longer accurate. Even census data, which is extensive and generally reliable, is a snapshot of a particular time. Since a full census is a once-a-decade event, census information may be as much as ten years out of date. There are updates in between, but only to selected categories and not every year.

5. Determine What Other Information You Need. Now is the time to finalize the questions you'll ask informants and the questions you hope to answer with the assessment. Those questions will depend on your purposes. In most cases, you'll want to determine what is important to population members or those who might benefit from or be affected by action resulting from the assessment. You will probably also want to hear the opinions of the people who serve or work with those people--doctors, human service staff and administrators, teachers, police, social workers, advocates, etc.

Before you start, take careful stock of your resources including people, money, skills, and time to ensure you can complete all plans. Many times, an assessment can be conducted with volunteers, or it may require statistical and other expertise including professional consultations. It is important NOT to plan an assessment without having resources needed to complete it.

6. Decide What Methods You'll Use to Gather Information. Here are some methods for gathering assessment data. They include:
- **Using Existing Data** – based on the information in census and other public records or to find information that's been gathered and recorded by other sources.

- **Listening Sessions and Public Forums** - "Listening" sessions are forums you can use to learn about how people feel about local issues and options. They are usually small with specific questions asked of participants that will give a sense of what the issues are and possible solutions. "Public forums" tend to be larger in number of participants and broader in scope than listening sessions. They are meetings where citizens can discuss important issues at a well-publicized location and time. It is an opportunity for people of diverse backgrounds to express their views, and it is a first step toward understanding the community's needs and resources.

- **Interviews and Focus Groups** - are less formal and conducted with either individuals or small groups (usually fewer than ten and often as few as two or three). They generally include specific questions, but allow room for moving in different directions, depending on what the interviewees want to discuss. Open-ended questions (those which demand something more than a yes or no or other simple answer), follow-ups to interesting points, and a relaxed atmosphere that encourages people to open up are all part of most assessment interviews. A focus group is a specialized group interview in which group members are not told what the interviewer wants to know so that their answers will not be influenced.

- **Observation** - Direct observation involves seeing with your own eyes how people use a particular area in their neighborhood, for example. It may involve participation on your part to really understand the culture and community.

- **Surveys** - can be a part of any or all of a community assessment. Written surveys may be sent to people in the mail, given out at community events or meetings, distributed in schools, or handed to people on the street. People may also be surveyed by phone or in person, with someone else writing down their spoken answers to a list of questions. Many kinds of surveys often have a low return rate and may not be the best way to get information, but sometimes they're the only way. They may be given in situations where most people complete them.

- **Asset Mapping** - focuses on the strengths of the community rather than the areas that need improvement. Focusing on assets empowers community members who directly experience the problem and already have the resources to change the status quo. If changes are made by the community and for the community, it builds a sense of cohesiveness and commitment that makes initiatives easier to sustain.

7. **Decide Where and From Whom You'll Gather Information**– it is important to get information from as broad a range of people and groups as possible. This will give you the real perspective of the needs and resources of a community, group, or individual. Of course, it depends on the specific purpose or goal; however, you do not want to miss valuable information. All viewpoints should be aired so there are no

surprises.

8. **Decide Who Will Collect the Data** – you might use members in the community to gather information or perhaps partner with a professional organization. The work of interviewing and surveying should be determined to find and collect data that can affect the quantity and quality of gathered information. Spend some time determining the best type of data gatherers to suit your plan of action.

9. **Decide How You Will Reach Your Informants** - To get information from people, they must be contacted. A more personal approach is often a more effective long-term approach. Using social media websites, such as Facebook and Twitter, are one option. Written surveys administered by telephone or emailed to organization-generated contact lists are also effective. Some organizations are willing to share their email lists. Short surveys in public places like shopping malls or sidewalks can be accomplished as well. Flyers and posters work well, or holding a press conference that appeals to existing community groups works well for reaching a large group. You might recruit friends, colleagues, neighbors, family members, etc. by phone or in person. They might also ask the people they recruit to ask others so that a few people can start a chain of requests that ends up possibly recruiting a large number of people.

10. **Decide Who Will Analyze the Data and How They'll Do It** – this means identifying the main themes from interviews and forums, sorting out the concerns of the many from those of the insistent few, understanding what your indicators seem to show, comparing community members' concerns with statistics and indicators, and perhaps a number of other analytical operations as well. You may need to hire a professional with knowledge of statistics and higher math, or it may require a common sense approach with the ability to group information in logical ways. If you hired a professional organization, they may want to be involved in the entire process from data collection to information analysis. It all depends on what kinds of information are needed to create a solid action plan.

11. **Plan Whatever Training is Needed** – this includes who will be involved and who will conduct the training. Training should be offered to all involved, even if some already have the skillset to do so.

12. **Decide How You Will Record the Results of the Assessment and Present Them to the Community** - Depending on your goals and what's likely to come of the assessment, "the community" here may mean the entire community or the community of stakeholders represented on the planning committee. In either case, you'll want to clearly explain what the assessment found and perhaps to help people strategize about how to deal with it.

Set out the results clearly, in simple, everyday language accompanied by easy-to-understand charts, pictures, and/or graphs. Your report doesn't have to be complicated or use technical language to be compelling. In fact, the more you use the words of community members who contributed their concerns and experiences, the more powerful your report will be.

With the availability of PowerPoint and similar programs, you have the opportunity to create a professional-looking presentation that can be presented as a slide show in one or more public meetings or smaller gatherings, posted along with a narrative on one or more social media sites (Facebook, YouTube, etc.) and/or on your website, run as a loop in a public place (like a local library), or even broadcasted on community access television.

13. **Decide Who Will Perform Which Assessment Tasks** – make sure that all tasks are covered and everyone has a role that fits his/her skills, preferences, and talents. Recruiting people should be part of the plan so needs can be anticipated. For example, if more people are needed for gathering data, then arrange to assign these tasks in the beginning.

14. **Create a Timeline for Assessments** - Create a schedule for the entire assessment process, including contacting people for training and preparing and printing surveys. Each part of the assessment process should have a deadline so you can finish the project in a timely manner and gather needed information.

15. **Present the Plan, Get Feedback** – Once the plan is completed, it may need to be adjusted to make it more workable. This adjustment will allow individuals to consider whether the plan considers the culture of the community and is likely to make data collection and analysis as easy as possible. As a result of feedback, parts of the plan can be adjusted to make them more acceptable to the community or more workable for the assessment team.

To get a comprehensive view of your situation in a group or community, it is important to look at what you have and what you need. Keeping these things in mind allows you to positively impact the problem you wish to address. Understanding a group or community's needs and assets will help clarify where to go and how to get there.

Training Different Populations
Training different populations can be challenging and may require training and structure. For example, Andragogy is a type of teaching strategy developed specifically for adult learners. It may be based on a humanistic conception of self-directed learners and teachers as facilitators of learning. It may be called "specific teaching methods" or "academic disciplines" or "adult education." Experience provides the basis for learning activities where adults must be responsible for decisions on education, planning, and evaluation of instruction. Most adults are interested in learning subjects relevant to their personal life or work and focus on solving problems, rather than just learning content. Andragogy allows discussion of the differences between 'taught' education and self-directed education and learning.

Learning Models

ARCS

This is an organization that recognizes the critical need for scientists and engineers in the United States. It invests in outstanding scholars who complete their degrees in science, medical research, and engineering. Scholarship awards are contributed through corporations, individuals, endowments, and designated all-women volunteer members to raise funds for the ARCS foundation. Many who have received their degree in these areas of study move on to enter the nation's government agencies and corporations to advance technology and science.

Gagne's Theory of Instruction

Gagne's Theory of Instruction is based on the fact that people's learning capabilities are broken down into several categories including learning verbal information, intellectual skills, cognitive strategies, attitudes, and motor skills. Each category leads to a different class of human learning performance. It considers previously learned capabilities and what is presented or given as instruction to the person learning. The goal of the theory is to promote the transfer of knowledge from perception through the stages of memory by first determining the objectives of the instruction. Each objective is stated using ONE standard verb, such as 'classifies' or 'states' or whatever is associated with a particular learning outcome. The instructor is then able to determine the conditions necessary for learning and incorporate that into the lesson plan or steps of instruction.

Bloom's Taxonomy

Bloom's Taxonomy is a classification of learning objectives and goals within education designed to improve communication among educators and the design of the curriculum including examinations. It is designed to promote the exchange of test materials and to stimulate research in relation between examining and education by classifying the goals of the education process. It includes classifying different objectives that educators set for students by dividing them into three areas: cognitive (knowing), affective (feeling from the heart) and psychomotor (actively doing something with the hands). Learning at higher levels is dependent on prerequisite knowledge and skills achieved at lower levels; however, the goal of Bloom's Taxonomy is to motivate educators to focus on all three areas to create a more holistic form of education. It is considered the foundation and essential element within the education community.

Maslow's Hierarchy of Needs

Maslow's Hierarchy of Needs is a theory proposed by Abraham Maslow in 1943 that extended the idea of including human beings' innate curiosity in describing the growth stages of humans. He used the terms *physiological, safety, love, esteem, self-actualization, belongingness,* and *self-transcendence* to describe the patterns that human motivations cycle through. As exemplary people, Albert Einstein, Frederick Douglass, Eleanor Roosevelt, and Jane Addams were studied rather than people considered mentally ill or neurotic who would yield crippled results (a popular framework used in sociology research and psychology).

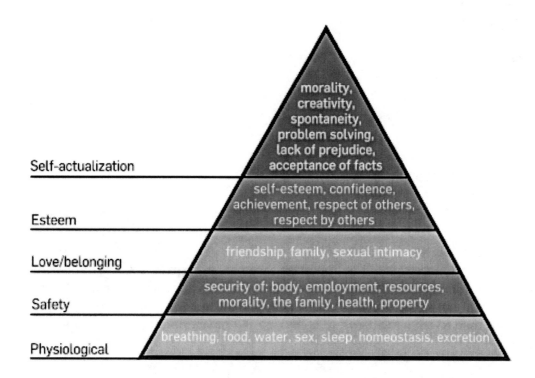

Existing Resources That Can Help Meet Training Needs

The assessment process greatly benefits from full community and stakeholder participation. Existing resources that can help meet training needs include:
- Those directly affected by adverse conditions and should be included in the planning process to meet those needs
- Individuals and organizations offering health and human services, especially those community-based with a strong connection to the populations they serve. They can be extremely helpful in sharing information, knowledge, and recruiting people who can contribute to the assessments and plans.
- Elected and government officials should engage in planning and carrying out assessments and training needs to ensure their success.
- Leaders in the community, such as directors of hospitals, college and university presidents, corporate CEO's, judges, doctors, and clergy who are known for their integrity, knowledge, intelligence, and good will.
- Professionals, such as police, teachers, emergency room personnel, and others who might be helpful when implementing new policies and procedures.
- Businesses that employ people from populations of concern or need whose lives might be affected by results of the assessments or plans.
- Community activists who have a stake in the planning of the assessment and who can address policies or issues that might come up during the process.

An Effective Training Plan

Once you have assessed and prioritized the need for training, the next step is to plan and deliver the training. The factors you'll want to consider include:

- Budget
- Training delivery
- Internal
- On-the-job
- Coaching
- Mentoring/buddy system
- External
- Professional seminars
- Private trainers
- Conference attendance
- Types of training

Impact on Business

Training costs money, and it is important to assess its impact in dollars and cents and determine whether the training is or was effective in reaching goals. Of course, changes will not occur overnight, so it is important to be patient and give the training program time to take effect before analyzing its impact on a business, community, or group.

Analyze Your Needs

When designing your training plan, take time to carefully analyze your needs. This analysis will help you choose the right type of training for your requirements. The strategic planning process incorporates many management practices, but also provides a methodical structure that can help you analyze your needs and make strategic decisions. Here is a step-by-step guide to analyze your needs and to plan a strategic process that will be effective and operational.

1. **Map Out the Present Situation at Hand** – Understanding where and what the current state of the organization, group, or community is in will help you understand strengths, weaknesses, opportunities, and threats that may be facing them. Conducting a communication audit will help you determine what strategies and activities are effective and where there is a need for improvement, with the available budget. One way to do this is to create a leadership survey that will help assess how much time, effort, and money is spent on specific activities and duties. This data will help determine gaps in performance and which tasks are most important.

2. **Talk to Key Stakeholders** – set up interviews with individuals and groups that will allow you to offer effective solutions and will help you understand more about what must be achieved. For example, in six months, what would you like to be different? Understand the current situation and look for roadblocks that might hinder program success. Who is directly affected?

3. **Be Clear About Your Vision for the Future** – envision what you want the program to look like, feel like, and operate like in one year's time. Outline specific details that all stakeholders can understand and support. What does success look like to you and to the organization, group, or individual? Ask stakeholders to write down as many ideas and concepts for each group or individual.

4. **Make a List of Priorities** – by identifying the most important aspects needed and by assessing current performance to get a clear picture of success from all key enablers for a successful execution of activities. What are the most important aspects for achieving the desired outcomes? Pursue all elements that appear critical or need improvement, first identifying the top three to six components.

5. **Develop an Action Plan** – that takes those top three to six elements and gives them specific 'end' points that provide an indicator of success and consider all resources, programs, products, and services that can help achieve each goal. Each objective must be S-M-A-R-T – specific, measurable, attainable, relevant, and time-bound. Assign individuals or groups responsibility for each objective, giving direction for developing a range of tactics and strategies to achieve each goal.

6. **Develop and Prioritize Potential Strategies and Tactics** – create teams that can brainstorm potential strategies to achieve each objective with specific methods and procedures for supporting each one. Strategies can be organized and consolidated with similar suggestions and voted on as to which are most likely to work and which might present difficulties. Determine which strategies to pursue and provide a clear direction with a designated time period for each one.

7. **Define Timelines and Responsibilities** – determine how success will be measured, the time frame allowed, and who will be responsible. For example, what is the desired outcome from the strategy? When should it begin and end? Which ones are urgent? Who and what is needed for success? There are four different types of measurable objectives including the financial impact, actions, audience perceptions, and communication activities. Through interviews and identifying what is currently known or believed to determine what changes or training must occur is key.

8. **Develop a Strategic Plan** – consolidate all ideas from each planning session and create a document with clear instructions and responsibilities for your team and other stakeholders for review and approval. Work with stakeholders and team members to clarify the specific details of each part of the plan and to map the results into a clear, detailed strategic plan.

9. **Put the Plan into Action** – implementing a plan is only the beginning of a long process of activities, measuring, reevaluating, and creating new strategies for success. Once a plan has been launched, determine regular review cycles for all phases, assessing all elements of the plan and their outcomes. Change the plan, if necessary, in response to changes in an organization, group, or other activities. Evaluating each individual's performance is critical for determining if some strategies should stay or be eliminated. Highlight areas that did not work including hurdles that prevented part of a plan or training from moving forward.

Serve as a Health Education Consultant

A health education consultant examines the efficiency, profits, and structure of an organization or group in the health education industry. After the examination is completed, a Health Education Consultant offers suggestions and strategies for improvement. A bachelor's or master's degree is required and certification is recommended. Some consultants are hired part-time while large companies that must find ways to improve or reorganize their health education programs may hire others full-time. Health education consultants may also develop a customer base on their own.

Duties include identifying problems that need to be fixed or changed by conducting preliminary research and examining current available data that is related to the problem or issue at hand. It may involve analyzing programs, revenue, employment numbers, and interviewing various people involved. A health education consultant can offer methods for improving a program's efficiency or for education and saving money. Once all research is completed, a health education consultant submits a written report to his/her client or organization contact where findings are discussed openly and a plan to implement changes is enacted.

The exact education requirements for a health education consultant vary based on an employer. Generally, the minimum amount of education needed is a bachelor's degree. Many employers prefer health education consultants with a master's degree, especially in private industries. Students interested in becoming health education consultants choose a major like management, marketing, economics, human resources, or business and a minor in health education or healthcare.

According to the U.S. Bureau of Labor Statistics, a health education consultant must be self-motivated and work with minimal supervision since employers expect them to be experts in improving an organization. Possessing effective communication skills is needed to clearly communicate improvement ideas with a client or group. The ability to handle stress and act responsibly is important, especially when health education consultants acquire more experience and are placed in charge of specific projects.

While certification is not a necessary requirement for this career, acquiring a Certified Management Consultant (CMC) designation can demonstrate an additional level of commitment to employers and customers. The Institute of Management Consultants USA, Inc. offers this designation to health education consultants who possess good references, have the required amount of education, complete an interview, and pass an examination (*www.imcusa.org*). To maintain this designation, a health education consultant re-certifies every three years.

Acting as Liaison
Health education consultants act as liaisons between different groups and individuals of an organization. They plan, implement, and evaluate health education programs in conjunction with local public health agencies and other providers. They develop criteria for on-site reviews of local health education programs to collect and analyze information necessary to evaluate its effectiveness, while consulting with administrators, legislators, media, and other interested parties.

Rules, policies, and procedures are developed for health education programs and services for implementation and establish contacts in public and private organizations. Evaluations are conducted in cooperation with program staff and help design health education and training programs for personnel and for state and local health agencies. A health education consultant develops educational materials, newsletters, reports, and other documents to enhance public awareness regarding health education programs. They also prepare requests for proposals, program agreements, and other materials to establish supported health programs and maintain all records and documentation related to the work completed.

Consultant Types

Health Education Consultant I
This is the training and first working level. Under close supervision, trainee incumbents will be trained to develop and strengthen skills in interpretation, application, consultation, and program planning in health education and will gain experience necessary to effectively perform at the first working level. Incumbents perform the more routine assignments and may assist in developing, monitoring, and evaluating established or new health education programs, projects, and policies.

Under supervision, at the first working level, incumbents also provide less complex planning, consulting, monitoring, and evaluating functions of health education policies, programs, and projects of average difficulty and related to a specific public health program; assist with more complex health education policies, programs, and projects; identify objectives and develop and evaluate program planning; participate in contract negotiations; select pre-testing methods and target groups; monitor program progress and contract compliance; participate in developing, coordinating, and conducting training programs; and coordinate inventory of educational resources and materials.

Health Education Consultant II
This individual is assigned a geographic area or special subject matter and works independently, providing complex health education consultation to private and public

agencies. They develop, plan, organize, monitor, and evaluate health education programs and projects while negotiating and recommending approval of contracts. A health education consultant (level II) develops, coordinates, and conducts training programs, serving as a leader to other health education consultants and staff. Developing and evaluating program standards, policies, and procedures is also part of this rewarding career.

Health Education Consultant III (Specialist)
Positions at this level are responsible for functioning as nonsupervisory technical specialists in the most difficult, complex, and/or sensitive programs and for making recommendations in policy development in their areas of expertise. Positions are allocated to this category when the level of expertise required is definably greater than at the journey level. Incumbents serve as highly skilled technical program education consultants or as recognized authorities in areas of extreme sensitivity and/or complexity. Incumbents have statewide responsibility for health education and related components of a major statewide project or program and may have coordinating or lead responsibility for health education and other professional-technical health staff.

The policy and/or program development responsibility at this level may significantly impact other departmental health programs or local, state, and federal agencies. The work performed at this level has the potential to establish new programs or majorly modify existing programs. Under general direction, incumbents provide the most complex consultation; develop, plan, organize, coordinate, implement, and evaluate the health education and related components of major statewide projects or programs; evaluate and ensure statewide program consistency; provide professional and administrative guidance to project staff in a lead capacity; propose and develop programs, legislation, regulations, policy, and procedures; and complete other related work.

Health Educational Consultant III (Supervisor)
This position is the first level supervisor. Under general direction, incumbents supervise a small to moderate group of health education consultants (three to seven). Incumbents may also have supervisory responsibility for a multidisciplinary health education administrative and clerical staff. Incumbents personally perform the most difficult, complex, or sensitive consultation, policy, and program development work.

Steps for Each Type of Consultation

The 'repeating' nature of the consultation process is essential, regardless of which stage of project consultation is occurring. The basic steps in the process will essentially remain the same and can be repeated as needed over the life of the project.

1. **Plan Ahead**
   Before beginning a stakeholder consultation process, it is useful to think about who needs to be consulted, over what topics, and for what purpose. Getting clear answers for these questions up front can save you time, reduce costs, and help

keep expectations realistic. For projects with multiple stakeholder groups and issues, it is recommended to prepare a more formal Stakeholder Engagement Plan in advance.

Stakeholder Consultation

Sometimes different organizations use different terminology -- be it "consultation," "public consultation," or "public participation" – to express similar concepts and principles. The core values of the International Association for Public Participation are as follows:

1. The public should have a voice in decisions about actions that could affect their lives.
2. Public participation includes the promise that the public's contribution will influence the decision. It promotes sustainable decisions by recognizing and communicating the needs and interests of all participants, including decision-makers.
3. Public participation seeks out and facilitates the involvement of those potentially affected by or interested in a decision.
4. Public participation seeks input from participants in designing the method through which they participate.
5. Public participation provides participants with information they need to participate in a meaningful way.
6. Public participation communicates to participants how their input affected the decision.

(Source: International Association for Public Participation, www.iap2.org)

For simpler projects and project expansions, it may be sufficient to verify that certain key questions have been considered. These questions may include the following:

- **Purpose** – What are the strategic reasons for consulting with stakeholders at this particular phase of the project? These activities may span a wide range of objectives that include meeting regulatory requirements and negotiating compensation to obtain access to community land for survey work, building trusting relationships, and managing expectations in general.
- **Requirements** – Are there requirements for consultation that must be met at this stage of the process? These may be legal or regulatory requirements, internal corporate policy requirements, or conditions of the lenders or shareholders.
- **Stakeholders** – Who are the key stakeholder groups that must be consulted during this phase of the project? What are the likely issues that they will wish to discuss? What are their interests and why?
- **Scoping of Priority Issues** – Are there any high-risk groups or issues requiring special attention at this stage? Are there vulnerable groups in the project area or topics that are particularly sensitive or controversial? Advanced planning may be required to tailor the consultation specifically to these needs.

- **Techniques** – Which techniques and methods will be most effective in communicating with the different stakeholder groups? Traditional or customary means of consultation and decision-making may be relevant here. Consider using participatory methodologies where appropriate and engaging skilled practitioners to facilitate the process.
- **Responsibilities** – Who within the company (or externally) is responsible for which activities? Are timetables, responsibilities, and lines of reporting for consultation activities clear?
- **Documentation** – How will the results of the process be captured, recorded, tracked, and disseminated?

2. **Conduct Consultations Using Basic Principles of Good Practice**

There is not one right way of undertaking consultation; given its nature, the process will always be context-specific. This specificity means that techniques, methods, approaches, and timetables will need to be tailored for the local situation and the various types of stakeholders being consulted. Ideally, a good consultation process will be targeted at those most likely to be affected by the project and be early enough to scope key issues that affect project decisions.

Relevant information that is disseminated in advance will allow it to be presented in a format appropriate for the group or individual. Both sides should have an opportunity to exchange ideas and information and also have their issues and concerns addressed. Keeping track of the key issues raised and reporting back to those involved in a timely manner clarifies steps throughout the life of the project.

3. **Incorporate Feedback**

Consulting entails an implicit "promise" that, at a minimum, people's views will be considered during the decision-making process. This promise does not mean that every issue or request must be acted upon, but it does mean being clear with people about which aspects of the project are still open to modification and which are not. It also means seriously considering feedback received during consultation and making the best efforts to address issues raised through changes to project design, proposed mitigation measures, or development benefits and opportunities. Inevitably, there will be limitations, both commercial and practical, in the degree to which stakeholder demands can be met. At other times, making modifications as a result of stakeholder feedback will make good business sense, will contribute to local development, or can be done as a gesture of good faith and relationship-building.

4. **Document the Process and Results of Consultation**

Documenting consultation activities and their outcomes is critical to effectively managing the stakeholder engagement process. When and where did such meetings take place and with whom? What topics and themes were discussed and what were the results? If commitments to stakeholders have been made during or as a result of these consultations, these too must be documented. The benefits of keeping such a record or "log" of stakeholder consultations are many. It may be part of ESIA regulatory requirements or valuable later in satisfying the due diligence inquiries of potential financial institutions and other equity partners.

Databases and Resources

A Health Risk Assessment (HRA) is a health questionnaire used to provide individuals with an evaluation of their health risks and quality of life. It incorporates three key elements that include an extended questionnaire, a risk calculation or score, and some form of feedback like a face-to-face session with a health advisor or an automatic online report.

The Centers for Disease Control define an HRA as: "a systematic approach to collecting information from individuals that identifies risk factors, provides individualized feedback, and links the person with at least one intervention to promote health, sustain function, and/or prevent disease."

There are a variety of different HRAs available; however, most capture information relating to the following:
- Demographic characteristics – age, sex
- Lifestyle – exercise, smoking, alcohol intake, diet
- Personal and family medical history (in the United States, due to the current interpretation of the Genetic Information Non-Discrimination Act, questions regarding family medical history are not permitted if there is any incentive attached to taking a HRA)
- Physiological data – weight, height, blood pressure, cholesterol
- Attitudes and willingness to change behavior to improve health

The main objectives of a HRA are to:
- Assess health status
- Estimate the level of health risk
- Inform and provide feedback to participants to motivate behavioral change to reduce health risks

Determining Reliability of Sources

The following principles should guide you in the collection, storage, and use of data for legitimate public health education purposes. A legitimate public health education purpose is defined as a population-based activity or individual effort aimed at preventing injuries, disease, or premature death. It also refers to the promotion of health education that includes assessing the health needs and status of a community or group through public health surveillance and research, developing public health policy, and responding to public health needs and emergencies. Public health purposes can include analysis and evaluation of conditions of public health importance and evaluation of public health programs.

The principles also reinforce data security standards defined here:

- Public health data should be acquired, used, disclosed, and stored for legitimate public health purposes.
- Programs should collect the minimum amount of personally identifiable information necessary to conduct public health education activities.
- Programs should have strong policies to protect the privacy and security of personally identifiable data.
- Data collection and use policies should reflect respect for rights of individuals and community groups and minimize undue burden.
- Programs should have policies and procedures to ensure the quality of data collected or used.
- Health education programs have the obligation to use and disseminate summary data to relevant stakeholders in a timely manner.
- Programs should share data for legitimate public health education purposes and may establish data-use agreements to facilitate sharing data in a timely manner.
- Public health data should be maintained in a secure environment and be transmitted through secure channels.
- Minimize the number of persons and entities with access to identifiable data.
- Program officials should be active, responsible stewards of public health education data.

Primary and Secondary Sources

Research that consists of collecting and organizing material from existing sources under provisions of this and other content policies is encouraged: this is "source-based research," and it is fundamental when writing an encyclopedia. However, care should be taken not to "go beyond" the sources or use them in novel ways. Sources may be divided into two categories:

1. A **primary source** is a manuscript, record, or document providing original research or documentation. A primary source is where original data, information, theories, or conclusions first appear, and all original research begins its life in a primary source.

2. A **secondary source** is a second-hand report or review of a primary source. It includes reviews or interpretations of original research and is written by someone other than the original researcher. A source may be both a primary source and a secondary source. For example, if a scientist reviews the experimental results of another scientist, his/her review is a secondary source. But if the scientist makes further novel conclusions based on the prior scientist's data, his/her writing is also a primary source.

   Secondary sources that review many primary and other secondary sources are sometimes called tertiary sources. This sub-category includes textbooks, treatises, dictionaries, and encyclopedias (such as Wikipedia). **Tertiary** sources are not usually sources of original research, though they may report and review original research found in other publications.

Written Resource Materials

What to Consider When Assessing Written Information

The ability to obtain, process, and understand written resource materials and information is essential for promoting and educating people and communities about health. Healthcare institutions and public health systems play a critical role in health literacy because they can make it easier or more difficult for people to find and use health information and services. National data demonstrates that currently available health information is too complex for average Americans to use to make health decisions.

Limited health literacy isn't a disease that makes itself easily visible. In fact, you can't tell by looking. Health literacy depends on the context. Even people with strong literacy skills can face health literacy challenges, such as when they:

- Are not familiar with medical terms or how their bodies work.
- Have to interpret numbers or risks to make a healthcare decision.
- Are diagnosed with a serious illness and are scared or confused.
- Have complex conditions that require complicated self-care.

Community needs can be defined as the gap between what is and what should be and can be felt by an individual, a group, or the entire community. It can be as concrete as the need for food and water or as abstract as improved community cohesiveness. Examining situations closely helps uncover what is truly needed and leads to future improvement.

Resources, or assets, can include individuals, organizations and institutions, buildings and equipment, or anything else that can be used to improve quality of life. For example, a farmers' cooperative that makes it possible for farmers to buy seed and fertilizer cheaply and to send their produce directly to market without a middle man, the library that provides books and Internet access to everyone, the bike and walking path where city residents can exercise all represent resources that enhance community life. Every individual is a potential community asset, and everyone has assets that can be used for community-building.

Online Information

Increasingly, consumers engage in health information seeking via the Internet. Health education professionals should be concerned about the topic, consider potential benefits, synthesize quality concerns, identify criteria for evaluating online health information, and critique the literature available online.

More than 70,000 websites disseminate health information; over50 million people seek health information online, with likely consequences for the healthcare system. The Internet offers widespread access to health information, advantages of interactivity, information tailoring, and anonymity.

However, access is not available to all, and use is hindered further by navigational challenges due to numerous design features, such as language that is too technical or a lack of permanence. Increasingly, critics question the quality of online health information as limited research indicates that much information is inaccurate.

Limited evaluation skills add to consumers' vulnerability and reinforce the need for quality standards and widespread criteria for evaluating health information. Existing literature can be characterized as speculative, comprised of basic how-to presentations with little empirical research. Future research needs to address the Internet as part of the larger health communication system and take advantage of incorporating existing communication concepts.

Not only should research focus on information quality, it also should address the quality of Internet use, on both an interpersonal and mass communication level, that creates avenues for investigation. We need to fully understand the influence of the Internet on health beliefs and behaviors including healthcare, medical outcomes, and the healthcare system.

Domain Name

The privacy of personal information, and health information in particular, continues to be a troubling issue in the United States. As more and more health information is computerized, individuals express concern about their privacy and that they are losing control over their personal health information. To help dispel public concerns, federal rules governing the use and disclosure of health information were promulgated under the Health Insurance Portability and Accountability Act (known as the HIPAA Privacy Rule). While the HIPAA Privacy Rule does not directly regulate researchers, it does restrict the manner in which healthcare providers may use and disclose health information for health research. Health researchers have been critical of the HIPAA Privacy Rule since its inception, concerned that it would interfere with valuable research. Various research organizations and others have requested that the law be revised to lessen its effect on research. Most recently, an Institute of Medicine (IOM) committee was formed and charged with reviewing the impact of the HIPAA Privacy Rule on health research.

Copyrights

Copyrights are original works of creative expression fixed in a tangible medium. Copyrights are exclusive rights, and the copying of a substantial portion of protected work or unauthorized use of protected work is an infringement of the owner's rights. As the National Institute of Whole Health has published over a dozen original handbooks, textbooks, manuals, and brochures, it is prohibitive in this limited space to identify all designated copy written material.

Priority Population

Well-planned health education programs incorporate collected data about the health issues addressed and other similar programs, plus they organize at the grassroots level to involve populations that will be affected. A health education program will be most successful if the priority population feels it has been instrumental in program development.

It is important to provide a sense of ownership and empowerment among those in the population of interest. Generally, the community organization process includes community recognition of the issue, entrance of health education specialists into the community to help organize citizens, community assessment, priority setting, selection and implementation of an intervention, and evaluation and reassessment of the action plan.

A Website's Appropriateness and Accuracy
There are a few things to consider when viewing health information on the Internet:

1. Sponsorship
Can you easily identify the website sponsor? Sponsorship is important because it helps establish the site as respected and dependable. Does the site list advisory board members or consultants? This detail may give you further insights into the credibility of information published on the site. The web address itself can provide additional information about the nature of the site and the sponsor's intent.

A government agency has *.gov* in the address, and an educational institution is indicated by *.edu* in the address. A professional organization, such as a scientific or research society, will be identified as *.org*. For example, the American Cancer Society's website is http://www.cancer.org. Commercial sites identified by *.com* will most often identify the sponsor as a company, for example Merck & Co., the pharmaceutical firm.

What should you know about *.com* health sites? Commercial sites may represent a specific company or be sponsored by a company using the Web for commercial reasons -- to sell products. At the same time, many commercial websites have valuable and credible information. Many hospitals have *.com* in their address. The site should fully disclose the sponsor of the site and the identities of commercial and noncommercial organizations that have contributed funding, services, or material to the site.

2. Is the Website Current?
The website should be updated frequently, especially since health information changes constantly when new information is learned about diseases and treatments through research and patient care. Websites should reflect the most up-to-date information and should be consistently available, with the date of the latest revision clearly posted. This date usually appears at the bottom of the page.

3. Factual Information
Information should be presented in a clear manner. It should be factual (not opinion) and capable of being verified from a primary information source, such as

professional literature, abstracts, or links to other webpages. Information represented as opinion should be clearly stated, and the source should be identified as a qualified professional or organization.

4. Who is the Audience?
The website should clearly state whether the information is intended for the consumer or the health professional. Many health information websites have two different areas -- one for consumers and one for professionals. The design of the site should make differentiating between the two areas clear to the user.

Reputable Affiliations
Evaluating reputable affiliations on the Internet has become more challenging. Anyone with the will and some computer knowledge can become his/her own Web publisher. Not only does this ability bypass traditional quality filters (like medical journal reputations, refereed review, and credentialed authors and editors) that we rely on for traditional journal literature, the electronic medium seems to offer information with a certain mystique that encourages many to accept it without question. It also tends to obscure some distinguishing characteristics that are often more obvious with print resources.

Without a healthy skepticism and set of evaluation criteria, the health consumer on the Web can be subjected to fraudulent claims and inaccurate information. Events have shown that the Web is a profitable haven for those promoting bogus and potentially harmful cures, drugs, and devices. The Federal Trade Commission, cooperating with the Canadian and Mexican governments, held a "Health Claims Surf Day" to ferret out dubious sites related to six diseases: AIDS, arthritis, cancer, diabetes, heart disease, and multiple sclerosis. Promoters and advertisers providing insufficient documentation were then notified that claims must be supported with reliable scientific evidence.

The World Health Organization established an ad hoc working group in late 1997 to develop recommendations to help regulate health ads and the sale of medical products, but the problems of these being adopted and enforced within a global computer network are daunting. The British Medical Journal recently reported that enforcement agencies from 20 countries searched the Internet for "potentially misleading health claims and miracle cures" and identified numerous bogus claims.

In addition to the problem of fraudulent claims is the danger of inaccurate or incomplete information from seemingly reliable sources. In one recent study, researchers surveyed the Web for parent-oriented health sites that provided information on managing a child's fever. 41 websites were identified, and 32 of them were commercial. The rest of the websites were from individual practitioners, clinics, and educational organizations. The information given at each site was compared with established treatment guidelines. Only one-tenth of the sites closely adhered to the guidelines. Several gave potentially harmful information like treating with aspirin. Many failed to provide complete information like how to take someone's temperature.

Physicians, teaching institutions, professionals, and health educators must take seriously the distribution and broadcasting of accurate information. They must warn their patients and clients about the need to critically review all medical information obtained from the Web, even when it seems to be from a 'reliable' source.

Web Evaluation Sites

The healthcare and library communities will continue to put mechanisms in place to evaluate websites. Currently, some Web directories provide "ratings" for sites, but a recent study of these found that less than one-third published their criteria. Of those that did, there was no indication of formalized evaluation addressing issues of reliability or construct validity. Several of the more notable Web directories with a health-specific scope include:

- American Medical Association Library Choices (www.amaassn.org/med_link/med_link.htm
- Health on the Net Foundation (www.hon.ch)
- OncoLink's Editors' Choice Awards (http://oncolink.upenn.edu/ed_choice/)
- Physician's Choice (www.mdchoice.com/)
- Six Senses Seal of Approval (www.sixsenses.com/)

Additionally, several sites exist that seek to identify problem websites. They include:

National Council Against Health Fraud (www.ncahf.org) – a non-profit and tax-exempt voluntary health agency that focuses its attention on health fraud, misinformation, and trickery as public health problems. It is private, nonpolitical, and nonsectarian. The organization is comprised of health professionals, educators, researchers, attorneys, and concerned citizens. Its officers and board members serve without compensation.

QuackWatch (www.quackwatch.com/) – "... a member of Consumer Federation of America, is a nonprofit corporation whose purpose is to combat health-related frauds, myths, fads, and fallacies. Activities include investigating questionable claims, answering inquiries, distributing reliable publications, reporting illegal marketing, improving the quality of health information on the Internet, and attacking misleading advertising on the Internet."

Evaluation Criteria

Beyond the guide and criteria offered by such Web directories, individual searchers— health consumers and professionals—must be prepared to judge the potential usefulness and reliability of information found on the Web. A set of common evaluative criteria is emerging from both the healthcare and library communities. The discriminating Web user should ask the following:

1. Who created the site?
- What is their authority?
- Do they have expertise or experience with the topic?
- What are their credentials and/or institutional affiliation?
- Is an email address provided for the person responsible for the site and/or its content?

- Is the site organization logical and easy to maneuver?
- Does the URL suggest a reputable affiliation with regard to the topic — personal or official site; type of Internet domain (*.edu*; *.org*; *.com*; *.net*; *.gov*; or *.mil*)?

2. Is the purpose and intention of the site clear, including any bias or particular viewpoint?

- Are the purpose and scope stated?
- Who is the intended audience?
- Is the information clearly presented as being fact or opinion and of primary or secondary origin?
- What criteria are used for inclusion of the information?
- Is any sponsorship or underwriting fully disclosed?

3. Is the presented information accurate?

- Are the facts documented or well-researched?
- Do the facts compare to related print or other online sources?
- Do the Web resources link to quality sites?
- Is the information and content current?
- Are the pages date-stamped with last update?

4. Is the site well-designed and stable?

- Is the site organization logical and easy to maneuver?
- Is the content readable by the intended audience?
- Has attention been paid to presenting the information without errors (e.g. spelling, punctuation) as much as possible?
- Is there a readily identifiable link back to the institutional or organizational homepage?
- Is the site readable by those with basic access capabilities (i.e. browsers and network speed)?
- Are links provided when necessary to download needed browser plug-ins?
- Is the site reliably accessible?

Applying the Criteria

Many sites will fail to sufficiently address all criteria. The searcher must approach each site with skepticism and with the intention of using the criteria to gather evidence of quality or lack thereof. These findings should then be substantiated by efforts to contradict or confirm based on other sources.

Finally, the purpose of the health consumer movement is to encourage individuals to be informed about best health practices and treatment options so that they are better prepared to make personal health decisions. The Web offers exciting opportunities for individuals to seek information to suit personal needs. It is the job of health professionals and librarians to emphasize that information learned on the Web must complement the communication between an individual and his/her healthcare provider.

Evidence-Based Strategies Available on the Internet

There is a way of providing health education that is guided by a thoughtful integration of the best available scientific knowledge and clinical expertise. This approach allows the health educator to critically assess research data, clinical guidelines, and other information and resources to correctly identify the problem, apply the most high-quality interventions, and re-evaluate the outcome for future improvement. The following are organizations and technologies that can assist a health educator in his/her endeavors:

NREPP

The National Registry of Evidence-based Programs and Practices (NREPP) is a searchable online registry of interventions that support mental health promotion, substance abuse prevention, and mental health and substance abuse treatment. Through NREPP, users can identify and learn more about interventions that may meet their needs. All interventions included in NREPP have been voluntarily submitted, have met a set of minimum requirements, and have been assessed by independent reviewers.

Electronic Mailing Lists

Electronic mail (email) is the exchange of text messages and computer files transmitted via communication networks, such as the Internet. Using an email system is the equivalent of postal mailing services, with the biggest difference being the time and cost involved. Email is not limited to written data; all sorts of information in the form of video, audio, or photographs can be sent via email. Email is an increasingly popular method of communication, especially in health education.

HEDIR

In 1992, Dr. Kittleson asked the chairs of the Health Education Programs at the American Association of Health Education's Annual Conference to forward emails from their colleagues so a directory could be created. Before that, he could send them out only one at a time. Soon an account was created by Southern Illinois University's Information Technology, and with one mouse click, the directory could be sent to everyone registered. An IT worker was asked to name the account, and he formulated an abbreviated name for Health Education Directory–HEDIR.

Today, over 2,000 members participate in HEDIR discussions, share information, or receive announcements on upcoming events. One can ask for assistance or ask a question and within minutes, he/she will receive at least 10 responses. HEDIR is responsible for creating the International Electronic Journal of Health Education, now owned by the American Association of Health Education. HEDIR continues to stay current and is the place for health educators to discuss a wide variety of topics online and receive responses from fellow colleagues.

Within the last few months, the HEDIR has teamed up with its long-time partner, HPCareer.net to organize and host a series of webinars. These webinars are free of charge and can be viewed online at www.healthpromotionlive.com. Additionally, individuals can earn CHES hours by attending live or watching the archived video and completing a series of assignments. HEDIR can also be found on Twitter, Facebook, and LinkedIn. The HEDIR will continue its efforts to use technology to encourage and train health educators. Eventual plans are to create an active HEDIR Wiki and HEDIR Second Life.

HEALTHPROM

This is an international development organization located in the UK that ensures that vulnerable children throughout Central Asia, Afghanistan, and Russia receive the best healthcare and education possible.

PubMed

PubMed is a free database offering the latest information on life sciences and biomedical topics and works closely with the MEDLINE database. The U.S. National Library of Medicine (NLM) at the National Institutes of Health used for retrieving information is responsible for maintaining PubMed. The drawback to this system is that MEDLINE uses terminology and vocabulary that you must be familiar with to understand the information presented.

The Medical Subject Headings (MeSH®)

The Medical Subject Headings (MeSH) is the authoritative list of the vocabulary terms used for subject analysis of biomedical literature at NLM. MeSH vocabulary is used for indexing MEDLINE journal articles and is also used for cataloging books and audiovisuals.

The MeSH-controlled vocabulary is a distinctive feature of MEDLINE that imposes uniformity and consistency to the indexing of biomedical literature, arranging the terms in a hierarchical categorized manner called MeSH Tree Structures. It is updated annually.

NCHS

The **National Center for Health Statistics (NCHS)** is a principal agency of the U.S. Federal Statistical System that provides statistical information to help guide actions, behaviors, and policies to improve health in the U.S.

NCHS is housed within the Centers for Disease Control (CDC) and is part of the U.S. Department of Health and Human Services (HHS). Headquartered in Hyattsville, Maryland, it offers data collection programs; conducts targeted surveys; and obtains information, such as birth and pregnancy rates and factors that affect them, adoptions, maternal and infant health; and supplements information for birth certificates collected through the National Vital Statistics System.

The State and Local Area Integrated Telephone Survey (SLAITS) allows them to produce state-level data on such topics as the health of children with special needs and to meet the data needs of our colleagues in HHS' Maternal and Child Health Bureau and elsewhere. They conduct the National Immunization Survey, in collaboration with the CDC, and periodically conduct longitudinal components to major ongoing surveys using the National Death Index that adds a lengthy component to their routine data systems. They develop and test data collection instruments for use in NCHS data collections and for surveys conducted by other federal agencies and research organizations.

HealthFinders

HealthFinders, Inc. is a nationwide recruitment firm that focuses on healthcare and pharmaceutical-related businesses. They specialize in the placement of healthcare professionals including executive management and field operational and sales personnel. Examples are Chief Operating Officer, Chief Nursing Officer, VP of Operations, VP of Sales, Regional or Area Directors, Director of Operations, pharmacists, medical sales representatives, sales executives, medical equipment sales, and marketing professionals.

They have over 60 years of experience in operations and sales management positions in those businesses. Their background includes knowledge of contract pharmacy and respiratory services to hospitals and long-term care facilities, contract research organizations, physician practice management, pharmaceutical companies, home care, and hospital management. The differentiating factors at HW HealthFinders are, and will continue to be, respect for the client's and candidate's time, understanding of the hiring manager's responsibilities, and the ability to match the appropriate candidate to the client's needs because of his/her extensive healthcare knowledge.

National Health Information Center

The National Health Information Center (NHIC) is a health information referral service that links people to organizations that provide reliable health information. The Office of Disease Prevention and Health Promotion (ODPHP), the Office of Public Health and Science, the Office of the Secretary, and the U.S. Department of Health and Human Services established the NHIC in 1979.

NHIC also supports the healthfinder.gov website, a reliable consumer health information source; however, it caters more to consumers rather than to professionals in the health fields.

GPO

Group Purchasing Organizations (GPOs) play a vital role in the U.S. healthcare industry. They help healthcare providers, such as hospitals, ambulatory care facilities, nursing homes, and home health agencies, save money by combining purchasing volume, using that leverage to negotiate discounts with manufacturers, distributors, and vendors.

A new survey finds that hospitals are generally happy with their arrangements, but cites certain limitations. During troubling economic times, cost control is crucial in the healthcare arena. Because supplies make up the second-highest expense in most hospitals, materials management has moved to the forefront of healthcare strategy. New health reform encourages providers to rein in expenses across all aspects of care. Hospital chief executives and chief financial officers are paying much closer attention to supply chain issues.

For decades, most hospitals and health systems have strategically managed their supply chains by using GPOs. These shared-service purchasing entities obtain volume discounts by combining the negotiating power of several hundred hospitals. In recent years, GPOs have expanded beyond their traditional roles to provide benchmarking data, consulting services, and quality monitoring. Hospital executives have long acknowledged that their GPO relationships bear value; although, how much value is still open to debate.

HON
Health on the Net Foundation (HON) is a not-for-profit organization founded in 1995 under the Geneva Ministry of Health based in Geneva, Switzerland. The organization came about following the gathering of 60 of the world's foremost experts on telemedicine to discuss growing concerns of the unequal quality of online health information. The unanimous conclusion of this gathering was to create a permanent body that would "promote the effective and reliable use of the new technologies for telemedicine in healthcare around the world." HON became one of the first organizations to guide both lay users and medical professionals to reliable sources of health information on the Internet.

SOPHE – Society for Public Health Education
SOPHE is a professional organization that was founded in 1950 to provide global leadership for health education and health promotion and to promote the health of all people by stimulating research on the theory and practice of health education. They support high-quality performance standards for the practice of health education and health promotion and advocate policy and legislation affecting health education and health promotion. SOPHE also develops and promotes standards for professional preparation of health education professionals and is the only independent professional organization devoted exclusively to health education and health promotion across all settings.

ASHA
The American School Health Association (ASHA) is the leading membership organization for school health professionals. It is concerned with health factors necessary for students to be ready to learn including optimum nutrition, physical fitness, and emotional well-being in a safe and clean environment. This broad spectrum of topics makes ASHA unique among health and education organizations and sets the stage for collaboration among its membership and partners.

Because of its diverse membership and proximity to Washington D.C., ASHA is able to collaborate and quickly respond to developments in the arena of school health. The visionary leadership of its board, staff, and membership makes the association a key figure in the effort to promote health for everyone learning and working in America's schools.

PHEHP
Public Health Education and Health Promotion (PHEHP) is one of 27 primary sections and special interest groups within the American Public Health Association (APHA) with over 3,000 members. Like all sections within APHA, PHEHP is governed by a group of elected volunteers who hold office for terms of varying length. Section officers include a chair, chair-elect, secretary, secretary-elect, and immediate past chair. Section counselors and governing counselors represent members and section concerns within the larger organization. A section committee, led by volunteers from the section, is where the "work" of the section is accomplished.

American Public Health Association (APHA)
This is a strong advocate for health education, disease prevention, and health promotion, directed to individuals, groups, and communities in all activities of the APHA. The organization's main goal is for all professionals and disciplines whose primary purpose is health education, disease prevention, and/or health promotion to set, maintain, and exemplify the highest ethical principles and standards of practice.

Education Resources Information Center (ERIC)
ERIC provides unlimited access to more than 1.4 million bibliographic records of journal articles and other education-related materials, with hundreds of new records added several times per week.

Within the ERIC collection, you will find records for:
- Journal articles
- Books
- Research syntheses
- Conference papers
- Technical reports
- Policy papers
- Other education-related materials

ERIC users include education researchers, teachers, librarians, administrators, education policymakers, instructors and students in teacher-preparation programs, parents, media and business communities, and the general public. The user community conducts more than 13 million searches each month through the ERIC website and commercial and non-commercial sites.

Children's Health Education Center
Children's Health Education Center offers resources and programs for children,

parents, teachers, and caregivers to help keep kids and teens healthy and safe. High-energy programs combine cutting-edge technology, engaging models, and hands-on learning for a dynamic, group-based educational experience.

CINAHL
Cumulative Index to Nursing and Allied Health Literature (CINAHL) is a database of over 3,000 nursing and allied health journals, evidence-based care sheets, quick lessons, CEs, books, dissertations, conference proceedings, standards of practice, software, and other references. You can get to the CINAHL from databases on the Lister Hill Library (LHL) website, and if you are having trouble finding what you are looking for, there is a librarian ready to help.

Evidence-Based Medicine Reviews (EBMR)
EBMR is a definitive resource for electronic information in the Evidence-Based Medicine (EBM) program that combines seven of the most trusted EBM resources into a single, easy-to-search database.

PsycInfo®
Currently, there are 2,521 journals in the PsycINFO® database. The list changes continuously as journals are added and discontinued throughout the year, so it is updated monthly online. You can download the journal coverage list as a Microsoft Excel file to see a list of currently covered neuroscience titles, journal coverage facts, and policies.

GEMS
The Graduate Education in Medical Sciences (GEMS) program is a structured educational experience for MIT PhD students interested in working at the intersection where engineering and science meet medicine and real-world healthcare. GEMS scholars learn how advances in basic science and engineering become medically relevant therapies and tools for the improvement of human health. GEMS graduates are well-prepared to become the next generation of leaders in medical-related research and biomedical business.

Their certificate program is open to doctoral students in MIT's Schools of Engineering and Science. It runs concurrently with the normal course of an MIT graduate education and can be completed in less than two years without prolonging a typical PhD education. In addition to coursework in pathology and pathophysiology, GEMS scholars attend seminars with HST students and participate in an individually tailored clinical experience. GEMS scholars develop lasting relationships with like-minded PhD students with complementary skill sets and with active physicians and physician-scientists.

The Institute for Medical Engineering and Science (IMES) offers GEMS through collaboration with MIT, Harvard Medical School, Massachusetts General Hospital, and Brigham and Women's Hospital. An award from Howard Hughes Medical Institute (HHMI) initially funded GEMS as part of a program to encourage graduate schools to integrate medical knowledge and an understanding of clinical practice into PhD curriculum.

Health Resources and Services Administration (HRSA)

This helps individuals not insured for healthcare; however, they can also help uninsured individuals get affordable health insurance coverage made available by the Affordable Care Act. About 1,200 health centers operate nearly 9,000 service delivery sites nationwide and serve approximately 21 million patients each year. Health centers have extensive experience providing eligibility assistance to patients and are providing care in communities across the nation.

With these new funds, health centers will be able to hire new staff, train existing staff, and conduct community outreach events and other educational activities. Health centers will help consumers understand their coverage options, determine their eligibility, and enroll in new affordable health insurance options. Community health center staff will provide unbiased information to consumers about health insurance, the new Health Insurance Marketplace, qualified health plans, and Medicaid and the Children's Health Insurance Program.

Funding received by the government allows the HRSA to align with other federal efforts, such as the Centers for Medicare & Medicaid Service-funded navigator program. Health centers work in communities across the country, which gives them a unique opportunity to reach the uninsured and help connect them with the benefits of health insurance coverage under the healthcare law.

AAHE

The mission of the American Association for Health Education (AAHE) is to advance the profession by serving health educators and others who strive to promote the health of all people through education and other systematic strategies. The AAHE addresses the following priorities:

- Develop and promulgate health education standards, resources, and services to professionals and non-professionals.
- Foster the development of national research priorities in health education and promotion.
- Provide mechanisms for the translation and interaction among theory, research, and practice.
- Facilitate communication among members of the profession, the general public, and other national and international organizations with respect to the philosophic basis and current application of health education principles and practices.
- Provide technical assistance to legislative and professional bodies engaged in drafting pertinent legislation and related guidelines.
- Provide leadership in promoting policies and evaluative procedures that will result in effective health education programs.
- Assist in the development and mobilization of resources for effective health education and promotion.

HaPI

Health and Psychosocial Instruments (HaPI) is a database that provides access to information, such as questionnaires, interview schedules, checklists, coding schemes, rating scales, etc. in the fields of health and psychosocial sciences, about approximately 15,000 measurement instruments. The full-text of the instruments is not included in the database; however, HaPI can be used to:

- Discover which instruments exist.
- Determine the availability of reliable and valid evidence.
- Track the history of an instrument over time.
- See which instruments have already been developed in your field of study.
- Locate ordering information for a known instrument.

The information in the database is abstracted from hundreds of leading journals covering health sciences and psychosocial sciences. Additionally, instruments from industrial/organizational behavior and education are included.

MedlinePlus

MedlinePlus presents interactive health tutorials from the Patient Education Institute where one can learn about the symptoms, diagnosis, and treatment for a variety of diseases and conditions. One can also learn about surgeries, prevention, and wellness. Each tutorial includes animated graphics, audio, and easy-to-read language.

Providing Health Information

Health Literacy

Health literacy is defined in the Institute of Medicine report entitled "Health Literacy: A Prescription to End Confusion" as "The degree to which individuals have the capacity to obtain, process, and understand basic health information and services needed to make appropriate health decisions."

Health literacy is not simply the ability to read. It requires a complex group of reading, listening, analytical, and decision-making skills and the ability to apply these skills to health situations. For example, it includes the ability to understand instructions on prescription drug bottles, appointment slips, medical education brochures, and doctor's directions and consent forms and the ability to negotiate complex healthcare systems.

Consequences of Poor Health Literacy

The relationship between literacy and health status in non-industrialized nations is well-known. Studies in these countries indicate a direct relationship between education level attained and key health status indicators, such as life expectancy and infant survival. Several studies conducted in the United States have confirmed that low literacy is directly correlated to poorer health and disease state outcomes. Consequences of inadequate health literacy include:

- Poorer health status.
- Lack of knowledge about medical care and medical conditions.
- Decreased comprehension of medical information.

- Lack of understanding and use of preventive services.
- Poorer self-reported health and compliance rates.
- Increased hospitalizations and healthcare costs.

Health Numeracy

When an educational booklet for diabetes states that "Even a small decrease in weight can reduce the chance of contracting diabetes," it may make sense to some people, but not to others. Even though there are familiar words in the sentence, readers must understand the quantitative meanings embedded in the words *small*, *decrease*, *weight*, *reduce*, and *chance*.

The term *health numeracy* indicates when individuals are able to access, process, interpret, communicate, and act on quantitative health information needed to be informed about health issues, perform routine healthcare actions, and make effective health decisions. Health numeracy includes a broad spectrum of quantitative concepts including some that are abstract (not concrete or visible). Risk and probability are examples of concepts that many people have trouble visualizing and understanding. Nonetheless, quantitative information is prevalent throughout healthcare and needed for tasks like measuring medication and calculating portion size. Here are some suggestions for clearly communicating health education terms:

Assume people lack knowledge of quantitative concepts. Many people, even those highly educated and literate, can have trouble understanding numbers or have an aversion to using them. While numbers may be second nature to scientists, the same is not necessarily true for all people and healthcare providers. Communicate to all in simple terms.

Focus on just one idea at a time. Many times, there are several quantitative concepts packed into one sentence. Focus on only one idea at a time and express it in simple sentences.

Offer support for ideas. Offer students support for learning new ideas. For example, draw a picture to convey an idea or use a physical representation of what needs to be conveyed with vivid language. Share a personal story to make ideas easier to understand.

Use numbers when they are needed. Even though numbers can be difficult to understand, sometimes, they are needed for precision.

Find out which measurement system is being used. In the U.S., most people are familiar with the customary U.S. system of measurement. But people from other countries likely use the metric system instead. Find out which system your student or client is familiar with and use it.

Dissemination

Dissemination means conveying or delivering a message to an audience at a variety of

155

different places. This process is the actual implementation of your health education activities. However, you should remember that health education is more than simply disseminating health education messages. To change behaviors, dissemination of your message should be accompanied by other supportive activities that facilitate the behavioral change process.

For example, you need to clarify misunderstandings, complement the content of your message with examples, and identify barriers that may prevent people from performing the beneficial behaviors. These actions may also involve providing resources needed to perform the health-related behavior, and it may be necessary to address cultural factors that may discourage the desired behavior.

Communication

The Master of Science in Public Health (MSPH) in Health Education and Health Communication program is designed for individuals seeking specialized formal academic training in health education, health promotion, and health communication. Fundamental skills and knowledge are necessary for careers in health promotion, education, and communication strategies and for working with individuals, organizations, and communities. Advanced skills in program planning, implementation, and evaluation are critical as are knowledge and skills for communicating health education concepts to an individual, a group, or a community.

Health Education Specialists

Health education specialists and public health educators are dedicated to promoting healthy behaviors necessary to reduce and prevent disease, injury, and disability. Their specific responsibilities include assessing individual and community needs for health education; planning, implementing, and evaluating effective health education programs; coordinating the provision of health education services; acting as health education resources; and communicating health education needs, concerns, and resources.

Key stakeholders for evaluations of public health programs fall into three major groups:
- Those involved in program operations: management, program staff, partners, funding agencies, and coalition members.
- Those served or affected by the program: patients or clients, advocacy groups, community members, and elected officials.
- Those who are intended users of the evaluation findings: program decision-makers, such as partners, funding agencies, coalition members, and the general public or taxpayers.

Clearly, these categories are not mutually exclusive; in particular, the primary users of evaluation findings are often members of the other two groups, such as individuals in program management or an advocacy organization or coalition. While you may think you know your stakeholders well, these categories will help you think broadly and inclusively when identifying stakeholders.

Potential stakeholders in public health programs include:
- Program managers and staff
- Local, state, and regional coalitions interested in the public health issue
- Local grantees of your funds
- Local and national advocacy partners
- Other funding agencies, such as national and state governments
- State and local health departments and health commissioners
- State education agencies, schools, and other educational groups
- Universities and educational institutions
- Local government, state legislators, and state governors
- Privately owned businesses and business associations
- Healthcare systems and the medical community
- Religious organizations
- Community organizations
- Private citizens
- Program critics
- Representatives of populations disproportionately affected by the problem
- Law enforcement representatives

Why Stakeholders Are Important to an Evaluation
Stakeholders can help (or hinder) an evaluation before it is conducted, while it is being conducted, and after the results are collected and ready to use. Public health efforts are complex and because public health agencies may be several layers removed from frontline implementation, stakeholders are particularly important in ensuring that the right evaluation questions are identified and that evaluation results will be used to make a difference.

Stakeholders are much more likely to support the evaluation and act on the results and recommendations if they are involved in the evaluation process. Conversely, without stakeholder support, your evaluation may be ignored, criticized, resisted, or even sabotaged. When reviewing the long list of stakeholders who might be generated in the three generic categories, using some or all of the evaluation standards will help identify those who matter most. It is important to prioritize stakeholders who:
- Can increase the credibility of your efforts or evaluation
- Are responsible for day-to-day implementation of program activities
- Will advocate or authorize program changes that the evaluation may recommend
- Will fund or authorize the continuation or expansion of the program

It is important to also include program participants and those affected by the program or its evaluation.

Responsibilities and Tasks of a Certified Health Education Specialist
As a Certified Health Education Specialist (CHES), you'll work with individuals and communities to improve or maintain their health by engaging in behaviors that promote positive health. You'll also be responsible for setting up and managing various programs intended to distribute information about exercise, nutrition, and disease prevention to those who need it.

It'll be your job to ensure that people receive health resources that most benefit them and suit their personal situations and cultural norms. Additionally, the National Commission for Health Education Credentialing (NCHEC) (*www.nchec.org*) cites seven key responsibilities of health educators:
- Assessing individual and community needs for health education.
- Planning health education strategies, interventions, and programs.
- Implementing health education strategies, interventions, and programs.
- Conducting health education evaluations and research.
- Health education administration and management.
- Providing health education resources.
- Health education communication and advocacy.

Education and Certification Requirements
To become a CHES, you must first receive a degree in health education, followed by an NCHEC certification. The degree must be in health education or a similarly related discipline that accurately and thoroughly covers the seven key responsibilities of health educators. The NCHEC requires at least a bachelor's degree for certification, but a master's degree is preferable by many employers and can lead to many more advancement opportunities. Receiving an NCHEC certification involves attempting and passing the multiple choice CHES exam that tests your knowledge of and competency in the seven key responsibilities.

Steps for Conducting Effective Presentations

Presentations take many forms. Some are extremely formal with highly detailed information, but how do you ensure that the audience doesn't get lost in the detail and lose focus of the overall message? Some are informal and make it difficult to control crosstalk among audience members.

What about the technical aspects? What will you do if the projector malfunctions? Do you have a backup plan? The desired outcome is that when the audience leaves, they will remember the information and be impressed with the overall presentation. Here are some steps and guidelines on how to accomplish just that:

Know Your Audience and Understand Its Perspective -- Whether your goal is to persuade, or simply to inform, you must understand your audience, its level of expertise, and how your message will resonate. Crafting a presentation for a group of high school interns would be very different compared to an executive report to management, pitching a sales idea, or addressing a hostile audience about why the company needs to cut benefits.

Do Your Research -- You absolutely must be an expert on your chosen subject. You don't need to be the world's leading authority on it, but you must know critical facts and much of the little-known information. Speaking about things everybody already knows about is a recipe for boredom. It's not unusual to spend weeks, or months, collecting facts, alternate opinions, and comments from reputable sources and thoughts of the general community.

Document Your Sources -- Where you get your information is as important as the information itself. Without solid, peer-reviewed data, you're just someone with an opinion. The audience, in this situation, is expecting facts and projections. Your personal opinion may very well be important, but it must not be the only information you present. The sources do not have to be listed; however, you should be able to give citations when asked.

Write Out Your Entire Speech -- This action does not mean you will read your speech word-for-word; however, it is important to be precise when speaking to the audience. If needed, print out the speech in large letters so you can glance at the words and know exactly where you are.

Prepare the PowerPoint Presentation -- If you're going to use a slide show, the visuals you show to the audience need to be designed to support what you're saying. Avoid too much detail; however, the title of each slide should reflect what you're saying or discussing. *Do not read the slide!* Assume the audience can read and let the visuals support your words, not duplicate them. There are very few things you can do that will have a worse impact than reading what the audience can read on their own. If all you're going to do is put up slides and repeat what's on them, then they don't need you.

PowerPoint slides, overhead projectors, blackboards, and whiteboards are "visual aids" and should be treated as such. First, they should be *visual*, focusing on graphics, illustrations, and plots rather than text. If your slides contain large blocks of text--or even a few sentences in bullet points--your audience will spend their time reading instead of focusing on you and the points you want to emphasize. Second, they should be *aids*--don't rely on the slides to make the presentation for you. Your speech should contain more content than the slides.

Avoid Packing Slides Too Densely -- If you put too much information up at once, the audience will lose focus. Keep your bullet points to around ten words or fewer.

Do NOT Use Too Many Flashy Graphics and Animations -- They divert attention from information on the slides and from *you*, the speaker, and what you are saying.

Time Your Presentation to Fit the Information -- If there is a time limit, be sure you don't exceed it and include time for questions, if that is planned. It is better to pare down the material rather than to rush through it more quickly. Time your visuals to coincide with your speech. Avoid unnecessary or redundant slides, such as outlines that describe the upcoming presentation. If you have more material than you can fit within the time limit, push that material onto "extra" slides after the end of your presentation. Those slides might come in handy if, during Q&A, someone asks for more detail. Then, you will look extra-well-prepared!

Make Sure the Color Schemes of the Slides Are Appropriate for the Presentation Venue -- In some situations, dark text on a light background looks best, while sometimes light text on a dark background is easier to read. You might even prepare a version of your presentation in both formats, just in case.

Rehearse Alone and Practice Often -- Read your speech and watch your presentation dozens of times. It needs to be so familiar to you that you know which slide is next, what you're going to say about each one, and how you will transition between slides… it must be second nature to you. When you begin to get completely bored by doing this and you know it from memory, then you're ready for the next step.

Do a Dress Rehearsal -- Enlist some people that you trust to give honest opinions. These should be people that are reasonably representative of your expected audience. Give them the whole presentation. Have them make notes during the rehearsal – where are you confusing and what is particularly good? Also have them concentrate on you-- are you moving around too much or too little? You don't want to appear "hyper," but you also don't want to come across as a monotone statue.

Tweak the Presentation -- Take what you learned in the dress rehearsal and make modifications. When you do this, try to put yourself in the audience's position. What will they hear when the slides are on the screen?

Prepare Yourself -- So far, the steps have all been about preparing your presentation. Now, it's time to think about you. Unless you do this for a living, you're going to be nervous. Visualize yourself in front of the crowd, doing a perfect job, and receiving applause. Find a quiet spot, close your eyes, and go over the presentation. Imagine yourself being completely in control and without stumbling. This is a very, very important step. Professional athletes use this virtually every time before they perform. It's a proven technique. Use it. You should also be doing this immediately before you go on stage.

Introduce the Presentation -- You've done a great job preparing, you know the material, you've rehearsed, and you've visualized perfection – in short, you're ready. One of the most important things you must notice is your physical demeanor. You don't want to look too stiff, and you don't want to look too casual. You should have already practiced the right stance and movement in your dress rehearsal.

Present the Material -- Remember, you are the expert. Methods to avoid "stage fright" vary from person to person (you have heard the advice to "imagine them in their underwear"), but one serious tip is to use eye contact. Present to one person, then another, and then another. Don't think of it as a large crowd--you're talking to one person at a time. Remember that YOU are the presentation.

Question and Answer Session -- This is optional, but can be an important way to clarify key points and be certain that your audience received your message. How to do a Q&A session is worthy of an article in itself, but there are a few things to consider. You must be in control. Some questions will undoubtedly be less than friendly. When you get those, answer them factually and move on. Just don't call on that person again.

You might get some "soft" questions that don't really ask anything new – be careful with those. They're easy and don't deserve a lot of time. Don't dismiss them or brush them off, but don't spend too much time rehashing what you've already said. Answer factually and perhaps bring in some new information, but then move on.

Open the Q&A with, "Before I close, are there any questions?". This question allows for a strong close and not a presentation that withers away with poor audience participation. When you're asked a question, first repeat it to the audience so everyone can hear it and then proceed to answer. Take a few seconds to formulate a clear answer before replying to a question. Failing to do so can lead to wandering or vague responses that do not reflect well on you as a speaker.

Exit the Stage Area -- Thank the audience for their attention and tell them the presentation is available in printed form. If you will be available for personal consultation, make sure you mention that. Don't spend a lot of time exiting; you're finished – exit graciously.

Event of Instruction
The American Association for Health Education has created topical resource sheets to help health education professionals identify and locate relevant information about health topics. Their mission is to advance professional practice and to promote research related to health and physical education including sports, dance, and other physical activities.

Chapter 7: Communicate and Advocate for Health and Health Education

Introduction
Health education specialists develop programs and services to improve the health of individuals and communities. Communication is essential to all phases of program development. Health education advocates work to empower individuals, make positive changes in the healthcare system, and improve access to healthcare. Since communication and advocacy are core competencies of health education specialists, preparation for the CHES exam must include knowing the roles of communication and advocacy in professional practice.

Creating Policies

Define "Policy"
The World Health Organization (WHO) defines health policy as "decisions, plans, and actions that are implemented to achieve specific goals within society." (1) Policies include laws, regulations, and rules. Policy interventions can be effective tools for health promotion and disease prevention, making it possible to affect chronic disease risks of many people simultaneously. (2)

There are several types of policies, including **broad-based policies, targeted laws, educational requirements**, and **community-wide interventions**. Examples of broad-based policies are the several bans and restrictions on smoking in public places. Child safety-seat laws are examples of targeted laws. Safety-seat laws target infants and children up to 4 years old.

Policies related to childhood vaccinations are examples of educational requirements. Vaccinations are required to attend schools and childcare programs. Water fluoridation policies are examples of community-wide interventions that affect entire populations in certain communities.

Factors That Affect Health-Related Policies
Health-related policies are influenced by a number of factors at the local, state, and national level. Policy is shaped by **existing policy and legislation**. Local politicians and state and national **legislators** are in the position to adopt and formulate policy and are considered key stakeholders in policy development. The need for health-related policy is unique in each community and depends on the **health status of the community** and the availability of **healthcare providers and services. Local business leaders, directors of organizations, funders, and clergy** can all play a role in influencing policy. The successful implementation of health-related policy relies on **identifying and engaging stakeholders.**

Access to **evidence-based research** can influence the decisions of governments or private sector groups to adopt certain healthcare policies. Evidence-based policy relies on research and the results of randomized, controlled studies to identify health programs that are effective and will improve health outcomes.

What Guides the Establishment of Health Program Priorities?
It is usually not feasible to address all health problems or issues of the community that are identified in the needs assessment. Establishing a process for identifying priorities is essential to ensure that resources are directed to the problems with the potential for the greatest impact on the health status of the community.

The process of prioritizing needs is best accomplished by a group of stakeholders who are familiar with the assessment data and are knowledgeable about the community. Establishing criteria and guidelines will provide a framework to help identify priorities. It is important that the individuals and organizations involved in the discussions understand and accept the criteria for recommending and adopting specific priorities.

Healthy People 2020 established national objectives that can serve as a starting point for identifying priorities. However, local and state priorities may differ based on the health status of the community. Before collecting new data about the problem, it is important to determine what data is already available. When gathering input to make priority decisions, it is important not to overlook additional sources of information in the community, such as:
1. Expert opinion
2. Public commentary about the problem
3. Results of opinion surveys

The Priority Rating System for Public Health Programs (PEARL) assesses the availability of interventions, the feasibility of implementing interventions, and the acceptability for addressing the problem or issue. (3)

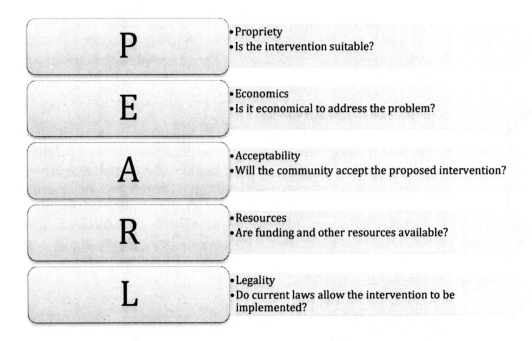

P
- Propriety
- Is the intervention suitable?

E
- Economics
- Is it economical to address the problem?

A
- Acceptability
- Will the community accept the proposed intervention?

R
- Resources
- Are funding and other resources available?

L
- Legality
- Do current laws allow the intervention to be implemented?

Other considerations for establishing priorities include:
1. **Impact of addressing the problem**
   If the needs assessment identifies a health problem, it is important to assess the feasibility and the potential impact of addressing the problem.
2. **Size or extent of the problem**
   Policymakers should determine the number of affected individuals and the seriousness of the problem. Consider the feasibility of implementing evidence-based interventions that will result in improved outcomes.
3. **Review best practices**
   For guidance on interventions, it is helpful to review current best practices that have been proven to be effective for a specific problem. Using others' experiences to address the problem will save time and resources.

Areas/Parts of Policy Development

Developing policy can seem like a daunting task. There are many areas to cover in the process. Following a policy development model helps divide the process into manageable steps and ensures that no essential parts of the process are omitted. Most policy models include the following stages: needs and resource assessment, agenda placement, policy formulation, implementation, and evaluation.

The first step of developing policy is to determine the current status of health outcomes, policies, and opinions. This step is followed by **agenda placement**. Agenda placement involves presenting the issue to a wide range of audiences. Audiences must be aware of a problem before they can become interested in working on solutions. A **needs and resources assessment** can effectively capture the attention of audiences. Community stakeholders can become involved at this stage to develop policies that address identified needs.

The next step in the process is to identify the legislative, judicial institution responsible for adopting and **formulating policy**. Stakeholders can offer expert guidance by providing scientific expertise and clinical experience in the community setting. Once a policy is established, health professionals in the community must implement it. Since the health professionals are familiar with the community, they are in an ideal position to work with local agencies to **implement health policy**.

Implementing a particular policy does not ensure that the health issue will be addressed. The policy must be evaluated to determine if it effectively solves the health problem it was designed to address. Community health workers and their colleagues are well-positioned to help **evaluate** the impact of policy changes. They can also mobilize continued support for policies that improve the health status of the community.

Key Steps of Policy Evaluation

The CDC developed a systematic framework to evaluate public health actions. The framework consists of steps in evaluation practice and standards for program evaluation. The framework emphasizes practical, ongoing evaluation strategies that involve all program stakeholders. Applying these framework elements ensures the development of effective programs and the continued improvement of existing programs. (4)

Standards are applied at every step of the evaluation framework. The four standards are:
1. **Utility**
   Utility standards ensure that the information needs of the evaluation users are met. They include identifying who will be impacted by the evaluation, the data that will be collected, the values used to interpret findings, and the clarity and timeliness of reports.
2. **Feasibility**
   The evaluation should use practical procedures and should acknowledge differing political interests of those involved. Resources should be used prudently and should result in valuable findings.
3. **Propriety**
   Propriety standards ensure that the evaluation is ethical. The evaluation must be conducted in a manner that protects the rights of program participants and evaluation users.
4. **Accuracy**
   The evaluation must produce findings that are considered correct. The purpose and methods of the evaluation must be described in detail. The evaluation should obtain data using systematic methods. Appropriate qualitative and quantitative methods must be used to analyze and synthesize the data. Finally, the evaluation report must be impartial and must contain justified conclusions.

Stakeholders are all the individuals or organizations involved in or affected by the program. Primary users of the evaluation are also considered stakeholders. Stakeholders must be engaged in the evaluation process to ensure that it addresses their concerns and values.

The **program description** conveys the mission and objectives of the program being evaluated. The evaluation must be descriptive enough to make the program goals and strategies understandable. The program description includes the following aspects:
1. **Need**
   A statement of need describes the problem being addressed and how the program will respond. Features of the program's need include the nature and magnitude of the problem, the populations affected by that problem, and whether the need is changing.
2. **Expected Effects**
   Program expectations state what the program expects to accomplish over time. The mission, goals, and objectives all address program expectations with varying degrees of specificity. The description of expected effects should also address any potential unintended consequences of the program.

3. **Activities**
   Activities specify what the program does to effect change.
4. **Resources**
   Time, talent, technology, equipment, information, and financial assets are all examples of resources.
5. **Stage of Development**
   Health programs mature and change over time. A program that was recently developed will differ from one that has been operating for over ten years. The program's maturity should be considered during the evaluation process.
6. **Context**
   The context includes the setting and environmental influences in which the program operates. It is essential to understand these influences to design a context-sensitive model.
7. **Logic Model**
   A logic model synthesizes program elements to visually present how the program will work. Logic models may be displayed as flow charts, maps, or tables to illustrate the sequence of steps leading to program outcomes.

A **focused evaluation design** ensures that the most-concerning issues are addressed without wasting time and resources. The following items must be considered when focusing the evaluation:
1. **Purpose**
   Public health evaluations have four general purposes: to gain insight, to change practice, to assess effects, and to affect participants of the evaluation process. The evaluation process may lead to organizational change and development.
2. **Users**
   Users are the individuals who will receive the evaluation results. User involvement clarifies the intended uses, prioritizes questions and methods, and assures that the evaluation remains relevant.
3. **Uses**
   Uses are the specific ways that evaluation findings will be applied. Uses should be planned and prioritized by the users.
4. **Questions**
   Creating evaluation questions encourages stakeholders to consider what the evaluation should answer. Questions help establish the evaluation's scope by defining which aspects of the evaluation will be addressed. Decisions about the questions will serve as a guide in subsequent steps of the evaluation process.
5. **Methods**
   Methods for the evaluation are based on scientific research of social, behavioral, and health sciences. The method may be experimental, quasi-experimental, or observational. Each method has its own bias and limitations, so evaluations that mix methods are generally more effective.

   Experimental designs use random assignment to compare the effect of an intervention with an otherwise equivalent group. Quasi-experimental methods compare non-equivalent groups. An example of a quasi-experimental design would be comparing program participants with individuals on a waiting list. Observational methods include comparative case studies and cross-sectional surveys.

6. **Agreements**

   Agreements describe how an evaluation will be implemented using available resources. Agreements clarify user roles and responsibilities. Aspects of the agreement include a statement of purpose, users, uses, questions, and methods. It summarizes deliverables, timeline, and budget. It can include stakeholders, but it should also include primary users and resource providers.

Gathering credible evidence provides a well-rounded program picture. Stakeholders should find the evidence believable and relevant. The information should answer stakeholders' questions and meet their credibility standards. Consulting an evaluation methodology specialist may be necessary if the concern for data quality is high or if there are serious consequences associated with making erroneous conclusions. Elements of evidence gathering include:

1. **Indicators**

   Indicators are criteria that will be monitored. Indicators include measures of program activities and program effects. Activities that can be defined and tracked include delivery of services, participation rate, and client satisfaction. Effects that can be measured include changes in behavior, health status, and quality of life.

2. **Sources**

   Individuals, documents, and observations are all considered sources of evidence for the evaluation. Selecting more than one source adds credibility to the evaluation. The criteria for selecting sources should be defined so that users can assess and interpret the evidence accurately.

3. **Quality**

   Well-defined indicators increase the likelihood of collecting quality data. Quality data is reliable, valid, and informative to evaluation users. Other factors affecting quality include instrument design, data-collection procedures, data collector training, data management, and routine error checking.

4. **Logistics**

   Logistics refers to the procedures for gathering evidence including timing, methods, and evidence handling. Procedures must be culturally sensitive and must ensure the privacy and confidentiality of evidence sources.

Justifying conclusions is an essential step to ensure that stakeholders will confidently use evaluation results. The process of using evidence to justify conclusions includes:

1. **Standards**

   Standards refer to stakeholder values. Those values provide a baseline for judging the program's performance.

2. **Analysis and Synthesis**

   Analysis isolates important findings, whereas the process of synthesis combines sources of information to reach a broader understanding. Mixed methods evaluations require both analysis and synthesis to accurately interpret the findings.

3. **Interpretation**

Interpretation is the process of determining what the evaluation means. Evaluation evidence must be interpreted to determine the practical significance of what has been learned.

4. **Judgments**

Judgments are statements about a program's worth or significance. Judgments are formed by comparing the findings to selected standards.

5. **Recommendations**

Recommendations are statements of actions to be considered based on evaluation. Forming recommendations is a distinct element in the evaluation process that requires information beyond what is needed to judge a program's merit. Even if a program is judged to be successful, it may not be recommended if effective alternatives exist.

Lessons learned from the evaluation do not guarantee that the findings will be used. Stakeholders and users must make a deliberate effort to ensure that the findings are appropriately used and disseminated. The five elements essential to ensuring evaluation use include:

1. **Design**

Design refers to how the evaluation is constructed. A design focused on use helps users know who will do what with the findings and who will benefit from being a part of the evaluation.

2. **Preparation**

Preparation refers to the steps taken to rehearse the eventual use of the evaluation. Preparation gives stakeholders time to explore potential positive and negative outcomes and to identify opportunities for program improvement.

3. **Feedback**

Feedback is the communication between stakeholders and users involved in the evaluation. Feedback can be encouraged by discussing each step of the evaluation process and by sharing interim findings.

4. **Follow-Up**

Follow-up is necessary to prevent lessons learned from being ignored or lost in the when making complex decisions. To ensure that this situation does not occur, someone involved in the evaluation should advocate it during the decision-making process. Advocacy increases the likelihood that actions will be consistent with the evaluation findings.

5. **Dissemination**

Dissemination is the process of communicating the lessons learned to relevant audiences. The communication should be timely, unbiased, and appropriate for the intended audience. The goal of dissemination is to achieve full disclosure and impartial reporting.

Framework for Policy Evaluation

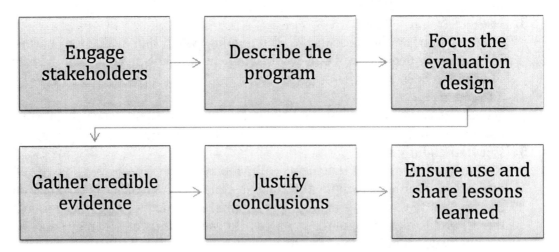

Resources

The Guide to Community Preventive Services is a resource for health educators and anyone interested in community health. The information provided in the guide is based on the scientific systematic review process. The guide is a collaborative effort by the Community Preventive Task Force and the CDC. Various partner agencies and organizations and individual policymakers, consultants, and researchers also help develop the guide. This resource is available at http://www.thecommunityguide.org/.

Health Education Advocate is a service of the Coalition of National Health Education Organizations (CNHEO). The coalition was formed in 1972 to expand and improve health education. The coalition fosters national communication between health educators and member organizations. Member organizations include Society for Public Health Education (SOPHE), American College Health Association (ACHA), American Public Health Association (APHA), Directors of Health Promotion and Education (DHPE), and American School Health Association (ASHA). More information about this resource is available at http://healtheducationadvocate.org/.

The Health Educator Job Analysis (HEJA 2010) was a national study describing the contemporary practice of health educators in the United States. The study was commissioned by American Association for Health Education (AAHE), Society for Public Health Education (SOPHE), and National Commission for Health Education Credentialing, Inc. (NCHEC). The purposes of the study included:

1. Validating the contemporary practice of entry-level and advanced-level health educators.
2. Guiding the development of the CHES and MCHES examinations.
3. Reporting the changes in health education practice since the previous job analysis study.
4. Developing professional preparation and continuing-education initiatives.

The national health educator Competencies Update Project (CUP) was initiated by NCHEC in 1998. The initial purpose of CUP was to determine the role of entry-level health educators by evaluating what they practiced. As a result of the findings of CUP, a three-tiered hierarchy was developed to define health educator roles at entry, advanced 1, and Advanced 2 levels of practice.

CUP research relates to the following three areas of professional focus:
1. Professional Preparation
2. Credentialing
3. Professional Development

Additional information about CUP research findings and recommendations are available at http://www.nchec.org/credentialing/competency/.

As professionals, health education specialists follow a **Code of Ethics**. The profession is dedicated to excellence in the practice of promoting individual, family, organizational, and community health. The Code of Ethics provides a framework of shared values within the profession. Professionals in all practice settings use Code of Ethics guidelines to assist in ethical decision-making. The seven articles of the Code of Ethics define specific responsibilities as follows:

- Article I: Responsibility to the Public
- Article II: Responsibility to the Profession
- Article III: Responsibility to Employers
- Article IV: Responsibility in Health Education Delivery
- Article V: Responsibility in Research and Evaluation
- Article VI: Responsibility in Professional Preparation

Health Communication

Goals and Components of an Effective Health Campaign

The CDC and the National Cancer Institute define health communication as "the study and use of communication strategies to inform and influence individual decisions that enhance health." (5) The **goal of health communication** is to promote health changes in individuals and communities using strategies based on science and consumer research.

Planning a health communication campaign requires knowledge of the health problem that will be addressed. Public health surveillance identifies the disease burden and specific behaviors, conditions, and policies that need to be changed. Research can help identify and prioritize the needs of the target audience.

The **major components** of an effective health campaign include:
1. **Describe the Problem**
   The problem is the main focus of the health communication effort. The description should clarify what the problem is, who it affects, and how it will be addressed. The problem analysis will help determine whether to pursue the effort.

2. **Perform Market Research**

   Market research is also referred to as consumer research. It is designed to increase understanding of the characteristics, attitudes, beliefs, values, behaviors, benefits, and barriers to behavior change in the target audience. The research helps create strategies for the health campaign.

3. **Define Market Strategy**

   A market strategy is a plan of action for the health campaign. The strategy includes the target audience segment, the behavioral change goal, the program's benefits, and the interventions that will influence behavioral change.

4. **Develop Interventions**

   Interventions are the methods used to facilitate behavioral change. Examples of interventions include holding training classes, developing a website, or expanding clinic hours.

5. **Evaluate the Plan**

   Planning the evaluation should be part of the planning process for the health campaign. The evaluation provides information about whether the program was implemented as intended (process measures) and whether changes occurred (outcome measures).

6. **Implement the Plan**

   The implementation component uses all planning and preparation completed in the previous steps. Activities include planning the launch of the program, holding a news event to publicize the program, taking advantage of unexpected opportunities, and neutralizing threats to the program. (6)

Health Communication Campaign Models

Communication is a transactional process and for health education professionals, it is an important aspect of their work. The communication transaction involves sharing information using a set of common rules.

There are numerous health communication theories, and no single theory is superior to another. Determining the theoretical model depends on the health education professional's personal choice, the target group, funding time, stakeholder influence, project size, and targeted behaviors. (7)

The two types of theoretical models are **cognitive theories** and **stage-step theories**. The **Theory of Planned Behavior (TPB)** and the **Health Belief Model (HBM)** are two examples of cognitive theories.

The TPB theorizes that the strongest determinant of behavior is the intention to perform the behavior. Intention is determined by the following three factors:
   1. Attitude to the behavior and balancing pros and cons associated with performing the behavior.
   2. Subjective norm, defined as the social pressure from significant others, such as peers, family, or media.
   3. Perceived behavioral control, or individual perception of the ability to perform the behavior.

The more positive the attitude, supportive the subjective norm, and higher the perceived behavioral control, the more likely the person will perform the behavior. The TPB has been successfully used to encourage walking among sedentary adults and to promote smoking cessation.

The Theory of Planned Behavior Model

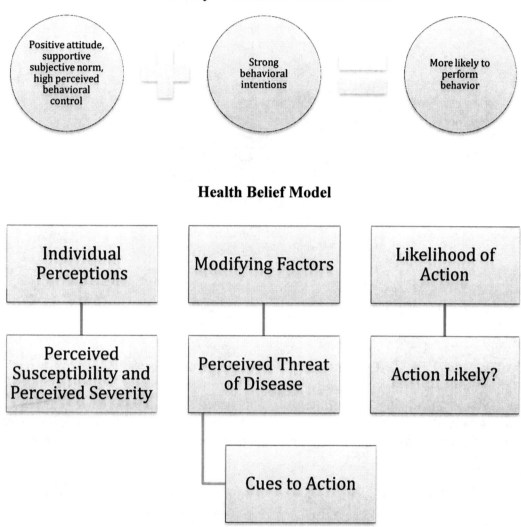

Health Belief Model

The **Health Belief Model** can be used as a pattern to evaluate or influence individual behavioral change. The model proposes that behavior can be predicted based on the degree of an individual's perceived vulnerability. Vulnerability refers to perceived susceptibility and the seriousness of the consequences. For behavioral change to occur, four conditions must be met:

1. The person must have an incentive to change.
2. The person must believe there is risk associated with continuing his/her current behavior.
3. The person must believe that change will have benefits.
4. The person must have the confidence to change his/her behavior.

Modifying factors are also important for behavioral change. These factors include demographic, socio-psychological, and structural variables that influence how a person perceives disease severity and susceptibility. Other important factors are age, gender, peer pressure, and prior contact with the disease.

The Transtheoretical Model

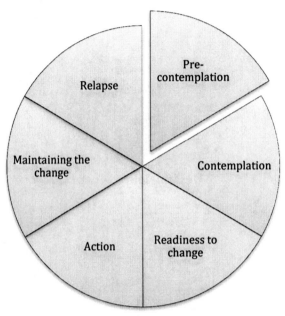

The **Transtheoretical Model (TTM)** is an example of a stage-step model. It is also referred to as the Stages of Change Model. This model proposes that people change their behavior at certain stages of their life. It is based on the premise that people are at certain levels of readiness to change. People move through various stages, but at any time, they may relapse and revert to previous patterns of behavior. A person may start at any stage in the model.

TTM was originally designed to promote smoking cessation efforts, but recently, the model has been used to promote fruit and vegetable consumption.

The Perceived Behavioral Control Model

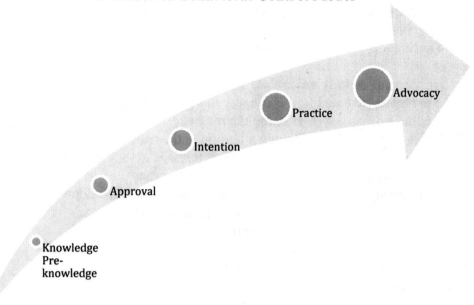

Another type of stage-step model is the **Perceived Behavioral Control (PBC) Model.** The main difference between this model and the TTM is that this model is not circular, but progresses upward in a series of steps until reaching the final goal. PBC was successfully used in efforts to persuade people to consume more calcium-rich foods. The following case study helps illustrate PBC in action:

1. Pre-knowledge
   The person is unaware they need to eat more calcium-rich foods.
2. Knowledge
   The person is aware that consuming calcium-rich foods will decrease the incidence of osteoporosis.
3. Approval
   The person is now in favor of eating more calcium-rich foods.
4. Intention
   The person wants to change his/her behavior to include consumption of calcium-rich foods.
5. Practice
   The person starts eating more calcium-rich foods.
6. Advocacy
   The person has been eating calcium-rich foods and now advocates his/her diet to others.

The Communication-Persuasion Model is different from other theoretical models because it is used primarily in the advertising field. The model is well-suited for use in mass media campaigns. The model can be characterized as an input-output matrix. The communication **input factors** include five separate stages of communication:

1. Source   Demographics, credibility, attractiveness, etc.

2. Message	Appeal, organization, style
3. Channel	Type of media used
4. Receiver	Demographics, social/psychological factors
5. Destination	Immediacy/delay, prevention/cessation

There are thirteen **output variables**, which must be completed in sequence for the message to be effective and for behavioral change to occur. The variables include:

1.	Tuning in	Hearing the message
2.	Attending	Paying attention to the message
3.	Liking	Liking, being interested in the message
4.	Comprehending	Understanding the message
5.	Generating	Thinking about what needs to be done
6.	Acquiring	Gaining skills to act on the message
7.	Agreeing	Agreeing that the message is correct
8.	Storing	Remembering the message
9.	Retrieving	Retrieving the message from memory
10.	Deciding	Acting on the message
11.	Acting	Performing the action
12.	Post-acting	Integrating the action into behavior
13.	Converting	Advising others to adopt the behavior

Stakeholders

Stakeholders are those who are affected by or are interested in a health campaign. Included in this group may be individuals who are interested in the campaign for academic, political, or philosophical reasons, but who are not directly affected by it. Based on their relationship to the health campaign, stakeholders may be further characterized as primary, secondary, or key stakeholders.

Primary stakeholders are people or groups who are directly affected by the health issue. Within this group of stakeholders, some may be negatively affected by a health policy, while others may benefit from the same policy.

Secondary stakeholders are people or groups who are indirectly affected, either positively or negatively, by a particular health policy. For example, a program to reduce the incidence of domestic violence may indirectly affect emergency room staff by reducing the number of abuse victims they treat.

Key stakeholders are influential people who can impact a health campaign. Examples of key stakeholders are organization directors, business leaders, legislators, funders, and clergy. (7)

Allies

Allies are the stakeholders who support the health campaign. They may be members of interest groups affected by the health issue, elected and/or appointed officials, or board members of local businesses who have a history of supporting related issues. An important strategy for recruiting and retaining allies is to involve stakeholders in every planning stage of the health campaign.

Use of Pictures

When pictures are linked to written or spoken words, they can increase the recollection of health education information. Pictures can also improve comprehension when they show relationships among ideas or illustrate special relationships. All patients can benefit from the use of pictures in health education materials, but individuals with low literacy are especially likely to benefit.

When used effectively, pictures help support key ideas in education materials, but health professionals should minimize distracting details in pictures. One effective strategy is to use people from the intended audience in the pictures. The effects of pictures can be evaluated by comparing responses to materials with and without pictures.

Culture

Culture can be defined as the shared knowledge, beliefs, and values that characterize a social group. Culture is also reflected in a group's norms, practices, communication patterns, and familial roles. (9) Culture is learned, shared, and transmitted from one generation to the next. Understanding the cultural characteristics of a given group can enhance the effectiveness of health communication programs and interventions.

Cultural competence refers to the ability to work effectively with individuals from different cultural and ethnic backgrounds. It includes the ability to understand the language, culture, and behaviors of other individuals and groups.

Cultural sensitivity is an aspect of cultural competence. It involves an effort from the health professional to be aware of and accepting of cultural differences. Cultural sensitivity also involves self-awareness of any biases or stereotypes.

To provide culturally appropriate programs and materials, health educators must understand how culture influences health behavior. Health educators can use several strategies to make health promotion programs and materials more culturally appropriate including:

1. Peripheral strategies

   Peripheral strategies are ways of packaging materials so they appeal to certain groups. This strategy can include using certain colors, images, fonts, and pictures of group members that are particularly relevant to the group.

2. Evidential strategies

   Evidential strategies emphasize a health issue's relevance to a group by presenting evidence of its impact on the group. This strategy is generally accomplished by using epidemiological evidence.

3. Linguistic strategies

   Linguistic strategies seek to make education materials more accessible by providing them in the primary language of the target group.

4. Constituent-involving strategies

   These strategies include hiring staff members from the target population and training paraprofessionals selected from the target group. Involving constituents can provide valuable insights into the cultural characteristics of the target group.

Material Distribution

Health education materials may be distributed in a variety of ways. The materials may be distributed by mail or in person. They may also be picked up from a rack in a health clinic, hospital waiting room, doctor's office, or community facility.

The distribution method will be determined by several factors including:
1. Whether the materials are intended to be used with or without the assistance of the health professional
2. Cultural preferences of the target audience
3. Type of health education material (e.g. pamphlet, factsheet, or booklet)
4. Topic of the material
5. Budget constraints
6. Preferences of the health education professional

Revising Material Based on Feedback

Revision of health education materials may be necessary to ensure that the materials are culturally sensitive and are understood by the target audience. Feedback from the target audience is obtained by pre-testing. The basic purpose of pre-testing is to determine whether readers understand the message.

Ideally, at least 25 to 50 members of the target audience should review the material. Pre-testing is usually completed when a rough draft of the material is available and again using a preliminary typeset, laid-out version of the product. Pre-testing can be completed in many settings including a client's home, a clinic waiting room, and a community center. If the material is intended to be distributed in a busy clinic, the pre-testing should be completed in the same setting.

Pre-testing can be administered to individuals or groups. It is important that participants understand that the product is being evaluated, not them. To ensure participants are comfortable criticizing the materials, reassure them that you want honest feedback. The people conducting pre-testing should be culturally sensitive and have good communication skills. Unless the potential participants feel comfortable with the interviewing staff, they may not agree to participate.

Literacy

Literacy is defined as an individual's ability to read, write, speak, compute, and solve problems at levels necessary to function in society. **Health literacy** refers to an individual's ability to process and understand basic health information and services needed to make informed health choices. (8)

Health literacy affects a person's ability to navigate the healthcare system. Health literacy is essential for an individual to share health information with providers, to manage chronic disease, and to understand the concepts of probability and risk.

Health literacy includes numeric concepts required to monitor blood sugar levels, measure medications, and compare insurance premium rates. People with low literacy may lack knowledge of how body systems work. They may have misinformation about the nature and cause of diseases. They may not understand the relationship between lifestyle factors, such as diet and exercise, and improved health outcomes.

Reading Level
According to the National Work Group on Literacy and Health, health education materials should not exceed the 6th grade reading level. Health educators must understand health literacy and readability to ensure that their education materials can be understood by the target audience. There are several tests and formulas available to evaluate the readability of health education materials including:

1. SMOG
   The SMOG Readability Formula uses a mathematical formula based on the number of words with more than three syllables (polysyllabic words). Sample sentences are taken from the beginning, middle, and end of a document. The SMOG formula is applied to all polysyllabic words found in the sample sentences. As an alternative to using the mathematical formula, the SMOG conversion table can be used to estimate the grade level of the text.

2. Fry Readability Formula
   The Fry formula is used to calculate the approximate reading level, or grade level, of a document. The formula is described as follows:

   Randomly choose three passages from the document and count exactly 100 words for each passage. Count the number of sentences in each of the three passages. Then, count the number of syllables in each passage. Divide by three to determine the average number of sentences and the average number of syllables in the three passages. The results are plotted on a Fry Graph to estimate the reading level.

3. Flesch-Kinkaid
   The Flesch-Kinkaid Grade Level Readability Score analyzes text and rates it based on the U.S. grade level. The rating tallies the average number of syllables per word and words per sentence. For health education materials, health professionals should aim for a score between 6.0 and 7.0.

   The Flesch Reading Ease Readability Score formula rates text on a 100 point scale based on the average number of syllables per word and words per sentence. The higher the score, the easier the text is to read. Health education literature should aim for a score of 60 or higher.

4. Gunning Fog Index
   The Gunning Fog Index Readability Formula is also known as the Fog Index. It is named after the man who developed the formula, Robert Gunning. The formula is applied to the number of words per sentence and the percentage of polysyllabic words to estimate the grade level of a document.

Audiences with Low Literacy
According to the 1992 National Adult Literacy Survey, approximately 90 million Americans, or 47% of the population, demonstrate low literacy levels. Literacy problems are present in all ethnicities, races, and classes. However, there is a significant correlation between literacy and levels of education and income. Many of the print materials disseminated by federal agencies are written at the 10th grade level or higher. These materials are not helpful to people with low literacy.

To develop effective print materials for individuals with low literacy, it is important to define the target audience. This task can be challenging since people with low literacy cross all ethnic and class boundaries. However, they do have some common characteristics in the way they process information including:
   1. Concrete versus abstract thinking
   2. Literal interpretation of information
   3. Insufficient language fluency to comprehend and apply information from written materials
   4. Difficulty with processing information, such as reading a bus schedule or a prescription label

To understand the physical, behavioral, and demographic characteristics of the target audience, it is essential to research the target audience. The research provides insights on what people already know about the topic, how they feel about the topic, and what information gaps exist. Research helps define the ethnic, cultural, and lifestyle preferences of the audience. This information is necessary to develop culturally relevant materials.

Existing sources of information about the target audience can be found in library databases, and health statistics can be obtained from local health departments. If there are gaps in the existing information, new research may be needed. Research methods include surveys, interviews, and focus groups.

The next step is to develop a concept for the product. This step involves defining the objective of the material. The objectives should be behavioral or action-oriented. It is essential to determine the key information the reader needs to achieve the desired objective.

For readers with low literacy levels, educational material should be written at an appropriate reading level so that the message is understood. Some experts suggest aiming for a reading level two to five grades lower than the highest average grade achieved by the target audience. Others state that a 3rd-5th grade level is appropriate for low literacy adults.

Types of Communication

Persuasive communication involves presenting arguments to motivate or change the audience. It is focused on changing the attitudes and behaviors of individuals and groups. As a health education professional, it is important to understand how to formulate a persuasive presentation. The key functions of persuasive communication are to:

1. Stimulate
2. Convince
3. Call to action
4. Increase consideration
5. Tolerate alternate perspectives

Stimulation involves presenting information that reinforces or intensifies existing beliefs of audience members. The process starts with identifying a foundation of commonly held beliefs and then presenting new information that supports the existing foundation.

Persuasive communication is **convincing**. The goal of a persuasive presentation is to change the attitudes, beliefs, judgments, and values of the audience. Although members may have their own beliefs and biases toward an issue, the goal is to persuade them to agree with the presenter's position.

A persuasive presentation has a **call to action**. The goal of the call to action is to persuade participants to change their behavior. The action may include **adoption, discontinuance, deterrence,** or **continuance**. As a result of listening to the presentation, participants may adopt a new idea or discontinue a negative health behavior. They may be deterred from starting a negative behavior if they have not already started it. Additionally, listeners may be motivated to continue healthy behavior.

Persuasive presenters are able to increase audience **consideration** of the presenter's point of view. While the participants may not be called to action, they may eventually be motivated to change their behavior.

Another aspect of a persuasive presentation is helping participants develop a **tolerance for an alternative perspective**. Developing tolerance for an alternative perspective may lead to increased consideration and an eventual call to action.

Electronic communication provides new tools for and new methods of communication. This form of interaction is interactive. It engages audiences in active, two-way communication. It also allows organizations to communicate quickly and inexpensively by using teleconferencing and videoconferencing.

Many organizations are using electronic communications, such as the Internet, as internal tools to enhance teamwork. Individuals at many locations can simultaneously work on the same documents, hold meetings, and discuss research findings. The Internet changes the way health educators can advocate positive health changes in the community. It provides new ways to inform legislators and influence public opinion about community health issues.

Top-down communication is a method of disseminating information within an organization using a hierarchical structure. Information originates from the highest-ranking members of an organization and filters down to the remaining members based on the organization's structure. It is essential that members in leadership positions know of their immediate supervisor and subordinate so that information is passed on efficiently.

The major advantage of top-down communication is that leadership controls the flow of information. A disadvantage of this type of communication is that some information may get lost in translation as it travels down the organizational hierarchy. Another disadvantage is that critical details of a project may be omitted if a high-ranking official forgets to include them in a report.

Communication Channels
The National Cancer Institute and the Centers for Disease Control and Prevention define health communication as "the study and use of communication strategies to inform and influence individual and community decisions that enhance health." (11) Health communication is a tool for promoting and improving the health status of individuals and communities. Successful health communication programs use research-based strategies to develop materials and to determine appropriate channels to ensure that those materials are delivered to the target audiences.

Interpersonal communication is a process used to communicate ideas, thoughts, and feelings between two or more individuals. It can occur face-to-face, by a person to an audience, over the telephone, or through email. The communication may be verbal or non-verbal. Non-verbal communication includes gestures, facial expressions, posture, and body language. It may be direct, as in face-to-face interactions, or indirect, as in computer-mediated communication.

The advantage of interpersonal communication, particularly face-to-face situations, is that people have an opportunity to discuss issues and receive immediate feedback. They also have the opportunity to evaluate non-verbal messages and relate them to verbal messages. They can also use the information to judge the credibility of the/a verbal message.

A major disadvantage of interpersonal communication is that non-verbal communication may be misunderstood when it occurs between people of different cultures. Differences in body language, eye contact, and meanings associated with gestures may all cause misunderstandings.

Community-based channels are used to reach a community, which may be a group of people in a geographic area or a group of people with shared interests. Examples of community channel tools include: community participation, community media, and community activities (such as fairs, conferences, and seminars). An advantage of community-based channels is that they can be specifically tailored to meet the needs of the target audience.

Organizational communication channels refer to the way that information flows within an organization and with other organizations. The flow of information is referred to as communication. In an organization, there are three communication channels: formal, informal, and unofficial.

Formal communication flows in a hierarchical pattern or top-down approach. Messages follow a chain of command. Managers pass information down to subordinates, and they pass the information down to the next level of staff. Examples of formal communication include policies and procedures, reports, and scheduled meetings.

An **informal** communication channel exists within an organization, but outside of the formal channel. Any communication that falls outside of the chain of command is considered informal communication. Lunchtime in the company cafeteria is a classic example of informal communication. Managers who adopt a hands-on approach and physically visit departments are using informal communication channels. Work teams are also examples of informal communication.

Some of the communication that occurs within an organization is interpersonal and relates to interests outside of the organization, such as sports and politics. The **unofficial** communication channel is also referred to as the organization's "**grapevine**." People who participate in grapevine discussions may form groups and develop friendships outside of the organization.

The advantage of using organizational channels is that they promote organizational efficiency, since management directs the flow of information. A manager skilled in balancing the three channels of communication may benefit from the advantages of organizational communication and may avoid potential pitfalls. There will always be a need for informal and unofficial communication channels within an organization, and balancing these channels effectively helps increase employee morale and team-building.

The disadvantage of using informal and unofficial communication channels is that there is potential to disrupt the chain of command, which may affect an organization's efficiency. At times, the influence of the grapevine may be positive, but often, information is exaggerated and rumors develop. It is essential that managers remain aware of the unofficial communication channel and make sure to dispel false information.

Newspapers are another form of mass media. Newspapers have a wide reach and may even target a global audience. The advantages of newspapers as a communication channel include accessibility and the ability to reach a specified target group. Newspapers tend to have a loyal following, which makes them desirable for advertising campaigns. Also, newspapers can be used for educational purposes.

However, there are several disadvantages to using newspapers as a communication channel. The information reported may not be authentic from every angle and may be misinterpreted. The news can be manipulated to influence audiences toward a particular point of view. The news articles may reflect the personal biases of the journalist or the editor. Also, newspapers have a short shelf life. From an advertising perspective, newspapers may not be an appropriate vehicle to promote certain products or messages.

Radio, a form of mass communication, is an effective method for broadcasting information to many people at once. Radio is an effective means of advertising, especially at the local level. One advantage of radio is that it is a relatively inexpensive medium for both the sender and the receiver. Radio messages may be prerecorded for a later broadcast, and receivers may record messages to listen at a more convenient time.

A disadvantage of radio is that receivers wanting to provide feedback about a particular message must use another communication channel (telephone, email, or letter) to respond to the sender. Also, since radio is generally used as background entertainment, receivers may pay less attention to the message than if it was delivered by another method.

Television, another form of mass media, is also an effective way to broadcast information to many people at once. Health education specialists can use television for educational programs and videoconferencing. Television can be used as a substitute for face-to-face communication because it engages auditory and visual senses.

An advantage of television is that it can replace face-to-face communication when time, distance, or travel cost would make face-to-face communication difficult. Since television combines audio and visual images, people can see non-verbal signals and listen to tone of voice to help interpret messages. Programs can be prerecorded and checked to ensure they communicate the intended message. People can also record programs to watch them at a more convenient time or to view them repeatedly so the message is understood.

The primary disadvantage of television is that it is expensive. The cost of equipment and videoconferencing rooms may be unaffordable for smaller organizations. It is also difficult to do well. It requires good cameras, trained operators, and an experienced producer. Also, individuals who appear on television must be trained to comfortably speak to a camera lens.

The **Internet** has grown exponentially in recent years. Most organizations have websites. The reason for the phenomenal growth of Internet communication is that it has many advantages of other communication channels and few of their disadvantages. Information presented on the Internet can include text, graphics, sound, and video. It can be prepared quickly and it allows immediate feedback. Some organizations design Intranet sites that are used exclusively by members.

The advantages of the Internet as a communication channel include:
1. Versatile use of text, graphics, animation, sound, and video to convey messages
2. Easy accessibility to individuals with an internet connection
3. Viewer ability to provide immediate feedback

The principal disadvantage of the Internet as a communication channel is that people must search for the information. The sender places the information on a website and then must wait for the receiver to access it.

Levels of Communication

Health communication programs effect change at many levels of communication including:

1. **Individual Level**

   Communication that occurs between two or more individuals occurs at the interpersonal level. This level is the most fundamental level of communication because individual behavior affects health status. Communication can affect an individual's awareness, knowledge, skills, and motivation to change health behaviors.

2. **Community Level**

   At the community level, policymakers can be effective allies to effect changes in policies and services. Through communication, they can advocate structural changes in the community, such as sidewalks, that encourage healthy behavior. Health communication can influence communities by promoting increased awareness of health issues.

3. **Social Network Level**

   A social network may consist of friends, colleagues, and other personal contacts. Having a strong social network can encourage healthy behavior. Examples of social networks include: exercisers at a gym, employees at a worksite, students and parents at a school, and patients and health professionals at a clinic. Activities aimed at this level take advantage of the strength of the social network to reinforce positive behavioral changes.

4. **Organizational Level**

   Organizations include businesses, associations, clubs, civic groups, government agencies, and health insurers. Organizations can support health communication programs. They can change policy to encourage positive individual health behaviors.

5. Societal Level

Health communication programs aimed at the societal level can change individual attitudes and behaviors. Society influences individual behavior by affecting norms, values, attitudes, and policies. For example, efforts to reduce drunk driving have changed individual and societal attitudes and behaviors. In this example, policy changes resulted partly from health communication at the societal level.

Health Marketing

Health marketing involves creating, communicating, and delivering health information and interventions using customer-centered and science-based strategies to protect and promote the health of diverse populations. (12) It is an innovative approach that draws from the fields of marketing, communication, and public health promotion. In its approach to promoting health to the public, health marketing blends theoretical principles of social marketing with outreach communication strategies of health communication.

Strategies

Health marketing strategies and techniques are based partly on traditional marketing theories. A market strategy is a guiding plan of action for a social marketing program. It includes the specific target audience, the desired behavioral change goal, the benefits of the behavioral change, and the interventions that support the behavioral change. There are ten strategic questions that can help develop a marketing plan. The questions are:

1. What is the social or health problem that must be addressed?
2. What actions will best address the problem?
3. Who is the target audience?
4. What does the audience want in exchange for adopting the new behavior?
5. Why will the audience believe that what is being offered is real and true?
6. What is the competition offering? Does the audience want what is being offered more?
7. When and where will the audience be most receptive to receiving the intervention?
8. How often and from whom does the intervention need to be received to be effective?
9. How can a variety of interventions be coordinated over time to influence behavior?
10. Are essential resources available to implement this strategy? If not, where can additional funding be obtained? (13)

Social Marketing

Social marketing is defined as the use of marketing principles to influence behavior to improve health or benefit society. (13) A principal feature of social marketing is its emphasis on bottom-up planning as opposed to top-down planning. Interventions are consumer-driven and are based on knowledge of consumer beliefs, needs, and perceptions.

Social marketing professionals identify the specific target audience, describe health benefits, and create interventions to support the desired behavioral change. Using research-based strategies, they aim to promote positive health changes in individuals and communities. Social marketing planning uses the "**4 Ps of Marketing**." They are:

1. Product
   The product may be a tangible object, a service, or a benefit of behavioral change. The product represents the desired behavior being asked of the audience.
2. Price
   The price is the cost of overcoming barriers faced by the audience when making the desired behavioral change. The cost may include financial, emotional, psychological, or time-related components.
3. Place
   The place is where the audience will access program products or services or where the audience will perform the desired behavior.
4. Promotion
   Promotion refers to the act of communicating the benefits of the program or product to the audience. It includes communication messages, materials, channels, and activities that will reach the audience.

A fifth "P" –Policy-- is sometimes included. Policy refers to laws and regulations that influence the desired behavior. An example of policy is the set of laws prohibiting smoking in public places.

Piloting and Revising Materials Steps
Piloting serves as a test or trial before implementing a health program. It is an effective way of ensuring that target audiences are responsive to the program and program materials. Pilot testing is performed to ensure that materials are effective and that the program is accepted by the community. Pilot testing may reveal sensitive issues that prevent acceptance of program interventions.

Basic steps for pilot testing and revising materials include:
1. Determine the Methodology for the Pilot Test:
   Methodology includes sample size and type of test. The test may be completed online, with pencil and paper, by telephone, in an individual interview, or in a focus group.
2. Develop a Checklist of Issues to be Addressed During the Test:
   Based on the issues identified, develop a list of questions to ask test participants. Feedback from test participants is recorded on the checklist tool during the pilot test.
3. Collect Feedback from Participants After the Test:
   Test results are compiled and analyzed to determine areas that need revision.

4. <u>Meet with the Planning Group</u>:
   During the meeting, decide which revisions should occur before launching the actual program.

Pre-testing occurs during all phases of development. Concepts, partially completed materials, revised products, and final products should all be pre-tested with individuals similar to the target audience. It is essential to understand how messages are perceived and interpreted by the target audience. Several rounds of pre-testing are required, but the benefits outweigh the time required for pre-testing, piloting, and revising material. Ultimately, the program will save time and money by getting it right the first time. Pre-testing allows health professionals to estimate audience response, to reduce the risk of disseminating the wrong message, and to develop effective materials.

Information Needs

Information needs of the target audience will vary depending on a number of characteristics, such as age, gender, education level, rural or urban location, culture, income level, and access to health services. Characterizing the target audience means determining essential traits, abilities, and knowledge of audience members. Characterizing the audience is an important step when planning health education programs.

What Are Information Needs Based On?
Information needs are based on an information needs assessment. This needs assessment allows health education professionals to tailor the message to the needs of the target audience.

Literature about information needs assessments recommends surveying 1-10% of the total population. In the surveys, it is helpful to include a cross section of the population. Some corporate leaders, change agents, and key stakeholders should be included in the surveys. Involving an influential person in the needs assessment may encourage participation and audience response.

Format options include written questionnaires, electronic questionnaires, face-to-face interviews, and focus groups. Key questions to use in the information needs assessment include:
1. What is the target population's knowledge of the issue?
2. Are they familiar with special terms and acronyms?
3. What type of training and skills related to the issue does the population have?
4. What tools and techniques are currently accessible to the population?
5. What are the personal benefits to the population to learn about the issue?
6. What educational methods will work best with the population?
7. Are there any cultural issues relevant to the population?

Factors that Influence Health Status
Individual health status is determined by circumstances and environment. Many factors combine to influence the health of individuals and communities. Some of the

factors that have the greatest impact on health include a person's home, a person's environment, genetics, income, education level, and social networks. To a lesser extent, factors like access and use of health services also influence health status. The factors and their influence on a person's health status are summarized as follows:

1. The higher the personal income, the better the health status will be.
2. Low educational levels are linked to poor health status.
3. Greater support from social networks is related to improved health.
4. Environmental conditions, such as clean air and water, healthy worksites, and safe housing, all contribute to good health.
5. Gender influences the types of diseases that affect individuals and the age when individuals will contract the diseases.
6. Inheritance plays a role in determining life expectancy and susceptibility to certain diseases. However, personal behaviors and coping skills also affect health status.
7. Accessing and using preventive health services will positively influence health status.

Pilot Testing

Pilot testing occurs before implementing a health education program. Pilot testing ensures that the program is effective and that members of the target population are responsive to it. The testing may identify culturally sensitive issues that may prevent implementation.

Advantages of pilot testing include:

1. Providing practical training for community educators
2. Testing the validity of education materials
3. Identifying areas that need revision
4. Improving the program and enhancing its performance
5. Preventing wasteful expenditures on large-scale programs

Major disadvantages of pilot testing include increased costs of program implementation and additional time spent conducting the pilot tests. Pilot testing can be conducted with a sample from the target audience or with a different audience similar to the target audience.

Methods

Pilot testing methods include using individual, face-to-face interviews; telephone interviews; and focus groups. Programs and materials may require several rounds of testing. Pre-testing occurs at each stage of development including:

1. Concepts
2. Partially completed materials
3. Revised products
4. Final products

Revisions

Revisions are based on the outcome of pilot testing. Revisions strengthen the overall effectiveness of the program. Several revisions may be required after each round of pre-testing.

Steps

The basic steps for pre-testing include:
1. Determining objectives
   Possible objectives include comprehension, attention-getting, relevancy, and persuasiveness.
2. Plan methodology
   Health education professionals develop test questions based on objectives and decide whether to conduct individual or group interviews.
3. Pre-test
   Interviews are conducted using test questions.
4. Revise, pre-test, revise
   Revision, based on data collected from interviews, occurs after each round of pre-testing.

Advocacy

Advocacy is a process to promote change in the policies, laws, and practices of influential individuals, groups, and institutions. It involves several individuals and/or organizations working together toward a shared vision of change. Advocacy for public health and for the health education profession is now considered an ethical responsibility.

Types of Advocacy

Interactive media advocacy uses the Internet and email in advocacy efforts. Social media is also a form of interactive web technology. Examples of social media include **websites, Facebook, Twitter, and blogs.** Interactive media allows users to find other users with similar interests. Users can join online communities to share information. Interactive media also provide opportunities for target audiences to contribute to advocacy campaigns.

Social media, such as Facebook, can be used to organize campaigns and build a support base. Each user has a webpage and profile, and users can comment on others' webpages. On Facebook, it is possible to:
1. Write short messages
2. Link to other websites and events
3. Post campaign photos and videos
4. Announce events and track attendees

YouTube is a website that hosts videos for users. In 2010, 85% of the U.S. Internet audience viewed online videos. YouTube can expand the reach of an advocacy campaign since the video will likely be viewed by a wide audience.

Blogs are informal online journals. They can be used to write about issues and policies. The blogs can showcase campaign successes, and photos and videos can be included. Blogs can also be used to post web links to other articles. Blog readers can comment on posts to communicate interactively.

Media advocacy is a type of health communication. It involves the ability of community members to be heard and to influence policy issues. One of the most powerful tools for community members to improve community health status is the mass media, especially the news media. Community groups can use media advocacy techniques to access the news media and advance public policy to enhance community health.

Media advocacy strategies include using focus groups and public polling to obtain information about what the target audience is thinking and to identify potential solutions to problems. The information is used to frame issues for the target audience. Community organization and coalition-building are also key elements of media advocacy. News strategies used by media advocates include establishing relationships with journalists, creating news stories, and using paid advertising.

Educational media is often used to educate individuals so they can make informed health choices. However, there are differences between education campaigns and media advocacy campaigns. Education campaigns inform or persuade the individual about a specific health issue and focus on individual behavioral change. The campaigns use various types of health communication approaches including mass media and interactive media. Contrastingly, media advocacy campaigns shift the focus from individual responsibility to social accountability. Media advocacy campaigns mobilize community activists and influence policymakers, and they also focus on changing the environment by changing policies.

Legislative advocacy involves working with legislators and legislative bodies to gain support for an issue and can involve meeting the needs of a specific population or organization. Successful legislative advocacy requires a well-organized advocacy group. Key steps in the process of legislative advocacy include:
1. Gathering allies
2. Designating a coordinator for the effort
3. Building a solid foundation about the issue
4. Defining the message
5. Creating an effective communication network
6. Establishing relationships with the media
7. Maintaining the effort for as long as needed

Policy advocacy is a type of legislative advocacy, but is concerned primarily with influencing public policy. It is defined as an effort to influence public policy by engaging in activities that encourage adopting the desired policy change. The focus of policy advocacy is on public policies and environmental changes that improve community health. Advocacy activities may include providing information, speaking to policymakers, and demonstrating the benefits of policy changes.

Proactive vs. Retrospective Advocacy

Proactive advocacy is the practice of looking ahead and preparing the organization or program for long-term success. Sometimes, it is possible to use advocacy to prevent a problem. Instead of waiting for an issue, such as a funding decrease, proactive advocacy involves outreach to key stakeholders and strategies to develop relationships and trust.

When a problem already exists, advocacy can be used to reduce it. This type of advocacy is referred to as **retrospective advocacy**. A common misconception about advocacy is that it must be adversarial between legislators and communities. However, most successful advocacy efforts involve building long-term relationships. Creating lasting change takes time and patience.

Components of Effective Advocacy and Developing Strategies

Voting-related behavior is a key element of advocacy efforts because voters determine elected officials and policymakers. Voting behavior strategies include registering to vote, encouraging others to vote, and serving as a deputy registrar.

Electioneering is defined as intervening in a campaign to support or oppose a candidate for public office. Public charities are permitted to lobby, but electioneering is prohibited. However, health educators acting as individuals can and do engage in electioneering activities. Strategies include contributing to a candidate's campaign fund, campaigning for a candidate, and seeking a political appointment.

Direct lobbying refers to attempts to influence legislation by communicating with legislators, staff, or other government officials. The communication must refer to specific legislation and reflect a perspective of it. Using this definition, a person who informs a legislator of his/her position on specific legislation is engaging in "direct lobbying." Strategies include contacting a candidate by letter, e-mail, fax, or phone. Meeting with policymakers is another excellent strategy. Health education professionals can increase their effectiveness by forming ongoing relationships with policymakers.

Grassroots lobbying is defined as efforts to influence legislation by attempting to influence the opinions of the general public. Grassroots lobbying must refer to specific legislation, reflect a perspective of it, and include a call to action. The call to action can include providing the name, address, or telephone number of a legislator. It can also include providing a copy of a petition or identifying a legislator's position on specific legislation. Grassroots lobbying differs from direct lobbying in that the legislator is not contacted directly and that there must be a call to action. Strategies include starting a petition drive, providing testimony at a policy meeting, and organizing a community coalition to advocate a health-related issue.

The Internet is a valuable tool for advocacy activities. It can be used to access and disseminate information about health issues. E-mail is also an effective way to communicate with policymakers and coalition members. Other Internet advocacy strategies include building a webpage about a specific health issue or policy and teaching others how to use the Internet in their advocacy efforts.

Media advocacy uses a wide range of strategies to advance healthful public policy. Focus groups and public opinion polling provide information about the causes and solutions of problems. Media advocacy involves building coalitions. Other strategies include cultivating relationships with journalists, creating news stories, linking issues with breaking news, and using paid advertising.

Sources

Many health education professionals do not believe they have the knowledge and skills to advocate. To gain confidence in advocacy activities, start with issues familiar to the health educator. Supplement knowledge with research about the specific issue and advocacy process.

The Internet is a powerful tool for conducting research about health issues and advocacy. **Health Education Advocate** is a website devoted to providing advocacy information to health education professionals. The website (**http://healtheducationadvocate.org/hea-summit/legislative-resources**) also lists resources and provides web links to agencies and education materials.

The APHA Media Advocacy Manual is a guide about how to use the media in advocacy campaigns. The guide provides tips for writing press releases and op-eds. The guide, developed by the American Public Health Association, can be downloaded from the Health Education Advocate website.

The Community Toolbox was developed by the Workgroup for Community Health & Development at the University of Kansas. Their website (**http://www.ctb.ku.edu**) offers advocacy tips and information about a variety of topics for health education professionals.

The Community Health Status Indicators Reports (CHSI) provides information about key health indicators for local communities. The reports were designed to be used by public health professionals and community members.

Research! America is a national not-for-profit agency for policy advocacy. Their website (**http://www.researchamerica.org**) includes legislative updates, talking points, and public opinion polls. The agency's goal is to obtain funding for medical and health research.

Moving Ideas, a website developed by the Electronic Policy Network, provides information and web links related to domestic and foreign policy and can be found at **http://www.movingideas.org**.

State and Local Government on the Internet is a website that provides web links to state and local government websites and to national organization websites. It can be found at **http://www.statelocalgov.net/index.cfm.**

The American Public Health Association website (**http://www.apha.org/legislative**) provides documents and web links related to legislative issues and advocacy.

Many national organizations, such as the **American Heart Association** and the **American Cancer Society**, are excellent sources of information about specific health topics. Health education professionals will select sources based on a particular health problem or issue of concern.

Five Elements to an Advocacy Plan

Advocacy must be based on solid planning principles. The planning approach used by media advocates is "GOTME"-**goal, objective, target, message, and evaluation**.

1. **Goal**

   Setting goals is an essential first step in any advocacy plan. When working with coalitions, it is especially important that each member clearly understands specific goals.

2. **Objectives**

   There are three levels of objectives involved in the advocacy plan. The first level is the overall objective that addresses what must happen to reach the program goal. The second level involves identifying specific policies that can be implemented to achieve specific objectives. The third level involves specific media objectives. Media approaches provide a powerful tool for achieving program goals and objectives.

3. **Target Audience**

   Media advocacy initiatives have three target audiences. The primary target audience is the person, group, or organization that can effect the policy change. The secondary target is groups or individuals who can be mobilized to pressure the primary target audience. The tertiary target group is the community.

4. **Message**

   There are at least three elements to the message. The first element is a clear statement of concern. The second element is the value dimension. An example of a value dimension is a potential threat to the welfare of the community. The third element describes the policy objective. Describing the policy solution is as important as describing the problem.

5. **Evaluation**

   The evaluation assesses the effectiveness of the advocacy program. It answers the question of whether the policy being advanced was actually enacted. The evaluation also assesses whether the issue became part of the media agenda. This detail can be determined by the amount of media coverage generated and the placement of that coverage.

The evaluation should assess whether the media coverage advanced the message. This detail can be determined by monitoring legislative progress and interviews with key advocates and decision makers. Polling community members is an effective way to determine if the issue reached prominence on the public agenda.

Implementing Advocacy Plan

Implementing the advocacy plan includes the following five steps:

1. **Getting the message across**

   Effective advocacy requires good communication. The message must be clear and compelling and should cater to the interests and knowledge of the audience. The message may be delivered as a written proposal, a face-to-face presentation, or a public demonstration. It also must be reinforced by repetition.

2. **Using the media**

   Advocacy initiatives use radio, television, newspapers, and online media. The media can increase the reach of an advocacy effort, but increased exposure also carries risks including mobilizing opposition to the program. Using the media requires skills in several media techniques, such as building contacts, writing press releases, placing stories, and organizing media events.

3. **Building partnerships and coalitions**

   Mobilizing public support is critical to the advocacy effort. Building partnerships and alliances are important methods for increasing a support base. Media and the Internet are essential tools for recruiting and maintaining public awareness of and support for the effort.

4. **Employing tactics and negotiation**

   Advocacy is a dynamic process, and it is important to maintain open communication. Policy and decision-makers may decide to respond to advocacy proposals with their own alternative proposals. Other interested parties may launch strategies to counter the original proposals. Because of these possibilities, it may be necessary to modify proposals to achieve results.

5. **Monitoring and evaluation**

   Monitoring and evaluation should occur throughout implementation. The process and results should be regularly evaluated during the program and after it ends to adjust strategies and the plan of action.

PhotoVoice

PhotoVoice is an organization that works globally with individuals, local communities, and partner organizations to create participatory photography programs. They build skills within disadvantaged and marginalized communities using innovative, participatory photography and storytelling methods. The program provides an opportunity for communities to self-advocate and effect positive social change.

Goals of the organization are:

1. To design and deliver tailor-made participatory photography, digital storytelling, and self-advocacy projects for socially excluded groups.

2. To bring together media, arts, development, and social change agendas to work on participatory photography and digital storytelling projects.
3. To work with communities on projects that give voice, build skills, provide advocacy platforms, and work towards sustainable change. (15)

Data

The data used to support policy change or an advocacy effort may be **qualitative** or **quantitative**. Qualitative data includes non-numerical observations collected in a systematic way using established social science methods. Quantitative data consists of numerical variables and statistics collected during the advocacy effort.

An important consideration when presenting data is to use it to develop clear messages. Dry facts and statistics can be turned into memorable messages. The data can be transformed into points that the target audience can relate to, such as sound bites or slogans.

Advocacy Evaluation Questions

A **formative evaluation,** or formative research, is conducted at the beginning of an advocacy program. The evaluation focuses on research that must be completed to develop the program. The **process evaluation** focuses on the procedures and tasks involved in program implementation.

An **outcome evaluation** examines program value to determine if short-term objectives were met. Contrastingly, an **impact evaluation** examines which long-term changes were achieved as a result of the program. An impact evaluation is the most comprehensive type of evaluation.

Basic process evaluation questions include:
1. Did the issue become part of the media agenda?
2. Was the issue framed from the policy perspective?
3. Did media coverage advance the message?

The final outcome measure is whether the policy was enacted. Outcome evaluation questions include:
1. Did the audience act as anticipated?
2. If the goal was met, which factors contributed to the intervention's success?
3. Is it possible to build on the program's success? How?
4. Should the program be continued?
5. If the goal was not met, how can the advocacy effort be improved?
6. Was the message clear?
7. Was the correct target audience identified?
8. Did the audience receive the message?
9. What is the next plan of action?

Models and Theories

Health Belief Model

The **Health Belief Model** is a psychological model that attempts to explain or predict health behavior. It was developed in the 1950s by researchers at the U.S. Public Health Service. The model attempted to explain why people sought x-ray examinations for tuberculosis. The model has evolved since then and has been applied to a variety of health behaviors. It can be used as a pattern to evaluate or influence individual behavioral change. The model proposes that the following four conditions explain and predict a health behavior:

1. People must believe they are susceptible to a specific disease.
2. People must perceive the "potential seriousness" of the disease in terms of pain or discomfort, time away from work, financial difficulties, and/or other outcomes.
3. People must believe the benefits of the behavioral change outweigh the costs.
4. People must receive a call to action or a precipitating force that compels them to change behavior.

Paternalistic Model

Paternalism occurs when a health professional makes a healthcare decision for a patient without his/her consent. In the traditional Paternalistic Model, the physician determined what to tell the patient about his/her diagnosis. In cases of a terminal illness, the patient was often not told about the nature of his/her illness. In recent years, the paternalistic model has been replaced by other models that emphasize shared responsibility and decision-making.

The **Paternalistic Model** is sometimes referred to as the parental or priestly model. In this model, the healthcare professional acts as the patient's guardian and determines which interventions will best promote the patient's health and well-being. The healthcare professional uses his/her knowledge and skills to determine the best treatment options and then presents them to the patient. The patient is encouraged to select the treatment plan that the physician has determined is best for the patient. In extreme cases of paternalism, the physician will authoritatively tell the patient which treatment will be initiated.

The healthcare provider has certain obligations in the Paternalistic Model. Physicians are obligated to prioritize the patient's interest over their own and to consult with other providers when more information is needed. In limited situations, the Paternalistic Model might be preferred, such as emergencies where the time required to obtain informed consent might have life-threatening consequences. However, in most instances, the preferred healthcare Provider-Patient Model is one that encourages shared responsibility and decision-making.

Scientific Model

This model is a basic element of the scientific method. It simplifies or substitutes for the topic being studied or predicted. **Scientific models** are not always complicated mathematical formulas. A good example of a scientific model is the USDA food pyramid. The model represents thousands of scientific studies on the relationships between diet, heart disease, and cancer. The model summarizes the findings in a picture that represents a healthy diet. It is a substitute for several scientific studies on diet and also for an actual diet.

The scientific method is a systematic process for conducting research and can be applied to many disciplines. The model for scientific research includes eight steps:

Identify the problem	• Develop a research question • Problem becomes the focus of the study
Review the literature	• Available research about the problem • Foundation of knowledge for researcher
Clarify the problem	• Narrow the scope of the study • Uses information from review of literature
Define terms and concepts	• Define terms as they relate to the study • Ensures that readers understand what terms mean
Define the population	• Focus on specific group of people • Narrows the scope to manageable size
Develop the instrumentation plan	• Road map for the entire study • Specifies who will participate and how, when, where data will be collected
Collect data	• Types of data: observations, questionnaires, literature • Data collected to answer research question
Analyze the data	• Determine if differences in data are statistically significant • Data analyzed to answer research question

Theory of Reasoned Action
The Theory of Reasoned Action is an example of a behavioral change theory. Behavioral change theories attempt to explain why behaviors change. The major factors in behavioral determination can be classified as environmental, personal, and behavioral characteristics.

The Theory of Reasoned Action assumes that individuals consider the consequences of a behavior before performing it. The theory uses two elements, attitudes and norms (or the expectations of others), to predict behavioral intent. Behaviors may be perceived as positive or negative based on the individual's views and on his/her impression of how society views the behavior. Intentions are shaped by personal attitudes and by social pressures. These intentions are essential to the performance of behaviors.

Theory of Planned Behavior

The Theory of Planned Behavior is another example of a behavioral change theory. It actually expands on the Theory of Reasoned Action. The theory proposes that the strongest determinant of behavior is the intention to perform the behavior. Intention is determined by the following three factors:

1. Attitude to the behavior and balancing pros and cons associated with performing the behavior.
2. Subjective norm, defined as the social pressure from significant others, such as peers, family, or media.
3. Perceived behavioral control, or individual perception of the ability to perform the behavior.

The more positive the attitude, supportive the subjective norm, and higher the perceived behavioral control, the more likely the person will perform the behavior. The Theory of Planned Behavior has been successfully used to encourage walking among sedentary adults and to promote smoking cessation.

This theory also emphasizes the importance of intention on behavior. However, it deals with cases where an individual does not control all factors affecting the actual performance of a behavior. The theory states that the incidence of actual behavior performance is proportional to an individual's total control over the behavior and to an individual's degree of intention to perform the behavior.

Public Service Announcements

Public service announcements (PSAs) are short messages developed to be aired on radio and television stations. PSAs are designed to persuade an audience to act. PSAs can be ready-to-air audio or video tapes, but some community stations prefer to receive a script that their announcer can read.

The format for writing a PSA includes the following guidelines:

1. The copy should be typewritten and double- or triple-spaced. Separate pages should be used for each 30-second spot.
2. The top of the sheet lists the duration of the PSA, the length of the PSA, the organization or group preparing the PSA, and the title of the PSA.
3. The script should be split into two columns. The left column lists directions, camera angles, and sound effects. The right column lists dialogue.
4. The bottom of the sheet should be marked with "###," indicating the end of the script.

Since time is limited in a 30-second spot, it is important to make every word count. The writing should be in plain language, and the message should be clear. The writing should use a "hook" to grab the audience's attention. The PSA should request a specific action, such as calling a phone number for more information.

Preparation is essential for writing and producing an effective PSA. The target audience and goals must be clearly identified. To best meet the needs of the target audience, the health education specialist should be aware of media outlet preferences of the target group. To approach media outlets, the health educator must be sure to contact either the station manager or the individual responsible for selecting which PSAs to broadcast.

Strategies for writing effective PSAs include:
1. Choosing one or two important focus points.
2. Brainstorming with colleagues and including members of the target group in the brainstorming session.
3. Checking facts to ensure the PSA is accurate and up-to-date.
4. Identifying a "hook" that will appeal to the target audience.

If the PSA will be pre-recorded and submitted to the station, it is recommended to seek external help to produce the PSA. However, it may not be necessary to hire a professional production company. Local advertising agencies or production companies may be willing to donate personnel, studio time, or equipment. Broadcasting students from local universities may also be a good source of talent.

Once the station agrees to broadcast the PSA, the health education specialist should contact the scheduler to find out when it will be aired. The health education specialist should watch or listen to the PSA to ensure that it was aired correctly. It is appropriate to send the station a thank you note and a small gift for running the PSA.

The best way to determine a PSA's effectiveness is to request a specific action and then monitor the actions taken. For example, if the audience is requested to call a phone number, then the number of calls received can be monitored before and after the PSA is aired. If the request is to attend an event, then attendance should be monitored, and the attendees should be asked where they heard about the event.

Test Your Knowledge

Chapter 1: Assess Needs, Assets, and Capacity for Health Education

1. True or False: Validity is how often an instrument accurately measures what it's intended to measure. Over time, if an instrument is unreliable and returns erratic results, it cannot be considered valid.

2. Reliability determines how consistently a measurement of knowledge or skill produces similar results under various conditions. If a measurement is highly reliable, it will yield consistent results over time. The way to estimate a measurement's reliability is:
   A. Inter-observer – is determined by how many different evaluators or observers examine the same presentation, project, paper, demonstration, or performance and agree on its overall rating.
   B. Test-retest – is determined by how often the same performance or test items evaluated at two different times yield similar results.
   C. Parallel-forms – are determined by examining how often two different measurements of skill or knowledge yield similar results.
   D. Split-Half Reliability – is determined by comparing half of a set of tests with another half and identifying how often they yield comparable results.
   E. All of the Above

3. Queries can be designed to pinpoint specific data elements across an entire population. The data is used to compile detailed reports that lighten the workload for case reviewers and ensure quality measurements with clinical documentation. Discrete data from narrations can be used to:
   A. Create patient or student action lists
   B. Add to electronic health records
   C. Target specific areas that need improvement
   D. Accurately chart reviews so only failed cases meeting query criteria are reviewed
   E. All of the above

4. Systematic reviews are designed to improve the cultural competence of health education professionals. Data is gathered before and after evaluations to compare and grade evidence as poor, fair, good, or excellent using predetermined criteria. There is excellent evidence that cultural competence training improves:
   A. Knowledge of health education professionals
   B. Attitudes and skills of health professionals
   C. Patient and student satisfaction
   D. All of the Above

5. True or False: The best approach for Mixed Methods Research is to yield efficient data collection procedures and facilitate group comparison within communities.

6. Formative evaluations provide information needed to adjust teaching and learning during an ongoing process. It allows students to measure their understanding during the learning process. The formative evaluation process guides teacher decisions about future instruction and programs. Examples include _____.
    A. Observations
    B. Asking questions
    C. Initiating discussions
    D. Graphic organizers
    E. All of the above

7. True or False: The Delphi method is a structured communication technique, originally developed as a systematic, interactive forecasting method that relies on a panel of experts. The experts answer questionnaires in two or more rounds.

8. True or False: "Asset Mapping" is not derived from an "asset-based" approach to community development. It refers to a range of approaches that work from the principle that a community can be built only by focusing on the strengths and capacities of the citizens and associations who call a neighborhood, community, or county "home."

9. True or False: Probability is a realization, or observed value, of a random value that is actually observed or is what actually happened in a given situation.

10. Examples of quantitative techniques include all of the following except _____.
    A. Surveys
    B. Questionnaires
    C. Pretests and post-tests
    D. Existing databases
    E. Statistical analysis
    F. Observations

Chapter 2: Plan Health Education

1. Which of the following is an appropriate learning objective?
    A. The health educator will demonstrate the correct use of a blood glucose monitor.
    B. The health educator will relate the benefits of a regular exercise regimen.
    C. The community will participate in a safety-oriented bicycle ride.
    D. The school age child will understand proper hand-washing technique.

2. Which teaching strategy is appropriate for the cognitive domain of learning?
   A. Discussion
   B. Role-playing
   C. Demonstration
   D. Practice

3. Which of the following aims to prevent the occurrence of health problems, disease, and dysfunction before it occurs?
   A. Primary prevention
   B. Secondary prevention
   C. Tertiary prevention
   D. Quaternary prevention

4. Repetition is one way that a teacher can help a learner with _____ barriers.
   A. Physical
   B. Sensory
   C. Affective
   D. Cognitive

5. Teaching methodologies must be consistent with the identified learning need, the domain of learning, the level of the domain, and the:
   A. Books that are used
   B. Learning objectives
   C. Style of teaching
   D. Learning styles

6. Which of the following stages of the group process focuses on decision-making?
   A. Forming stage
   B. Norming stage
   C. Storming stage
   D. Negotiation stage

7. Which of the following is an example of a well-worded learning objective of the psychomotor domain?
   A. At a second first-aid class, the student can answer questions regarding information learned in the first class.
   B. After a CPR class, the student is able to tell a friend what CPR stands for.
   C. After a CPR class, the student is able to explain how to perform CPR.
   D. After a CPR class, the student is able to perform CPR.

8. Sensory barriers to learning can be eliminated with:
   A. A comfortable ambient temperature
   B. An open and trusting environment
   C. Large print materials
   D. Clarification and re-clarification

9. Educational content should be sequenced according to movement from the:
    A. Simple to the complex
    B. Threatening to the non-threatening
    C. Psychomotor domain to the cognitive domain
    D. Unknown to the known

10. Which fact about culture is accurate?
    A. People within a culture share a common physical characteristic.
    B. People cannot have more than one culture, each with its own beliefs.
    C. Culture and ethnicity are essentially the same concepts.
    D. Cultures have their own vocabulary and terminology.

11. An ethical concern for health educators is:
    A. Teaching in an honest, fair, and respectful environment
    B. The need to coerce clients into making better health-related choices
    C. The need to eliminate communication and collaboration among learners
    D. Discrimination and a failure to make reasonable accommodations

Chapter 3: Implement Health Education

1. Which of the following is NOT one of the Five Phases of Implementation?
    A. Establish a management system
    B. Enact the plans
    C. Administer program evaluation
    D. End or sustain the program

2. An example of a behavioral objective for a health education program might include which of the following?
    A. After completing the program, 80% of participants will express the intention to begin a new exercise regimen.
    B. After completing the program, 80% of participants will report an increase in the number of exercise sessions they participate in per week.
    C. Half of all program participants will attempt a new physical activity.
    D. By the six-month follow-up, half of all program participants will remember the weight loss techniques discussed during the intervention.

3. Which type of intervention involves promoting a change in policy or public action on behalf of a particular group?
    A. Advocacy interventions
    B. Behavioral interventions
    C. Educational interventions
    D. Service interventions

4. What is the name of the committee commonly in place to review the ethical design of a study or intervention?
    A. Intervention Review Council
    B. Institutional Review Board
    C. Ethics Evaluation Committee
    D. Committee for Ethics Review

5. In what primary, significant way does pretesting differ from pilot testing?
    A. Pretests allow comparison with a post-test for program evaluation; pilot testing is a complete evaluation of the program.
    B. Pretesting tests a portion of an intervention before complete implementation; pilot testing involves a complete run of the program, but with only a small segment of the target (or similar) population.
    C. Pretesting involves gathering data on program participants at the beginning of an intervention; pilot testing involves gathering data about program acceptability from a population without the same need for the program as the priority population.
    D. Pretests allow the health educator to tailor information to particular program participants; pilot tests allow the health educator to discuss program material in a focus group with potential participants.

6. Which of the Four Ps of Marketing should be considered when scheduling the intervention or delivering the program?
    A. Price
    B. Place
    C. Promotion
    D. All of the above

7. Which of the following models would lead a health educator to implement intervention activities that promote self-efficacy?
    A. Health-Belief Model
    B. Logic Model
    C. Precaution Adoption Process Model
    D. Transtheoretical Model

8. Which of the following factors is unlikely to be a significant problem with program materials distributed to intervention participants?
    A. The brochures are written at a health literacy level that does not match the target population.
    B. The brochures include photographs of individuals who do not represent the culture or demographics of the target population.
    C. The brochures include graphics or colors that do not match the formality level of the other aspects of the program.
    D. The brochures include too much information and inadequate white space, making them confusing or uninteresting to the target population.

9. Gantt charts differ from task development timelines in what primary way?
    A. Gantt charts include a second line indicating task progress compared to expected task duration; task development timelines do not.
    B. Gantt charts allow separation of tasks by type or staff member; task development timelines do not.
    C. Gantt charts always color-code task importance; task development timelines do not.
    D. Gantt charts use calendars for a visual representation of task organization; task development timelines do not.

10. When implementing a health education program, an excessive monetary incentive may violate which ethical principle or concept?
    A. Non-maleficence
    B. Autonomy
    C. Informed consent
    D. Proportional risks and benefits

Chapter 4: Conduct Evaluation and Research Related to Health Education

1. Select the type of research that is accurately paired with its characteristic.
    A. Qualitative—Deductive
    B. Quantitative—Inductive
    C. Qualitative—Null hypothesis
    D. Quantitative—Null hypothesis

2. The purpose of a review of the literature is to provide researchers with:
    A. A critique of the research before it is used
    B. A fuller understanding of the topic of interest
    C. Validity and reliability statistics for their study
    D. The basis for justifying the research

3. An example of a null hypothesis is:
    A. Performance levels will increase over 3 days of night shifts.
    B. Compliance rates will decrease as illness severity increases.
    C. The clients will have an increased quality of life after education.
    D. Compliance rates will not increase after education.

4. Which sample will lead to poor research results?
    A. A sample that is large
    B. A sample that is too small
    C. A random sample
    D. A sample consisting of only females

5. Reliability reflects a measurement tool's ability to:
   A. Measure what it is supposed to measure
   B. Avoid extraneous variables
   C. Avoid intervening variables
   D. Measure the variable consistently

6. Validity reflects a measurement tool's ability to:
   A. Measure what it is supposed to measure
   B. Avoid extraneous variables
   C. Avoid intervening variables
   D. Measure the variable consistently

7. The most commonly used scale for research is the _____.
   A. Guttman Scale
   B. Likert Scale
   C. Yes/No Scale
   D. Multiple Choice Scale

8. Which of the following is an example of a central tendency used to analyze quantitative data?
   A. Multiple regression
   B. T-test
   C. Median
   D. Chi-square test

9. As you are reading a research study, you see that the hypothesis was supported at p < .10. What does this mean?
   A. The results have less than a 10% chance.
   B. The results have less than a 90% chance.
   C. The results are 10% reliable.
   D. The results are less than 90% reliable.

10. Qualitative research data is analyzed by:
    A. Using descriptive statistics
    B. Using inferential statistics
    C. Critiquing soundness
    D. Searching for patterns and trends

Chapter 5: Administer and Manage Health Education

1. Health education can occur in a variety of settings including insurance companies, medical clinics, foundations, and health associations. It can also be provided in:
   A. Hospitals
   B. Universities and colleges
   C. County, state, and federal government services
   D. Nursing homes and assisted living places
   E. All of the above

2. True or False: Maintaining integrity in the promotion and delivery of health education is the key to respecting the dignity and rights of all people served.

3. The essential elements for developing and maintaining a successful, effective partnership are:
   A. Mutual trust and respect – establishing a relationship in an effective partnership within an organization and/or the community is an ongoing process.
   B. Agree on a mission, goals, values, and objectives that serve the organization and community and that yield high quality services in all programs. It is important to realize that changes prioritizing the community over the program may be necessary for best results.
   C. Balance power and share resources with all partners involved. Balancing power is the key to a successful, thriving relationship and prevents misunderstandings. This balance may be difficult during times with limited resources and diverse communities and may involve control over grants or real estate issues, for example. Moderating the imbalance of resources and promoting a shift towards attaining common goals helps represent all partners involved.
   D. Openly communicate with partners and develop a common language. Recognizing differences at the onset of a partnership and reminding everyone of common goals can help prevent the end of a potentially productive relationship.
   E. All of the above

4. True or False: A health education leader must possess a positive attitude and be able to coordinate a variety of tasks and responsibilities, using appropriate time management skills.

5. Define the terms MOA and MOU.

6. True or False: Age Discrimination in Employment Act (ADEA) means it is unlawful for an employer to refuse to hire or to discharge anyone with respect to compensation, conditions, terms, or privileges of employment due to age.

7. The importance and objectives of an external assessment include:
   A. A degree or certificate
   B. Comparing abilities
   C. Evaluating an institution's progress
   D. Attaining employment for selection of intelligent educators and employees
   E. All of the above

8. When evaluating qualifications during the interview process where appropriate questions and issues are addressed to evaluate prospective health education professionals, what should be noted when asking, "What type of education/training does the candidate have?"
   A. Graduation date, all degrees, and type of specialty certification
   B. Titles of continuing education courses completed in the last 2 years
   C. Where and when licensed, registered, or certified (ask for documentation)
   D. Years of experience in occupational health
   E. All of the above

9. True or False: The FIRST STAGE of team developing involves forming a team that meets and learns about the opportunities and challenges, agrees on goals, and begins to tackle the assigned tasks.

10. Team-building activities help improve communication between members by helping them understand each other, can boost morale, and are effective learning tools to improve productivity and performance. Learning each other's strengths and weaknesses promotes better teamwork for increased success. Team-building activities include:
    A. Problem solving
    B. Decision-making activities
    C. Building trust
    D. Communication
    E. All of the above

Chapter 6: Serve as a Health Education Resource Person

1. A health education resource person educates people about health and includes both individuals and groups of people for promoting, maintaining, and restoring good health. The profession involves the following areas of health:
   A. Environmental
   B. Physical
   C. Social
   D. Emotional and Spiritual
   E. Intellectual
   F. All of the Above

2. True or False: The responsibility of each health educator is to aspire to the highest possible standards of conduct and to encourage the ethical behavior of all his/her colleagues.

3. True or False: Policies, programs, and priorities should be developed and evaluated through health education processes that ensure an opportunity for input from community members.

4. True or False: A foundation, including those of charities, is a legal classification or category of non-profit organizations that usually donate funds and support other organizations through charitable means.

5. Gagne's Theory of Instruction is based on the fact that people's learning capabilities are broken down into several categories including:
    A. Learning verbal information
    B. Intellectual skills
    C. Cognitive strategies
    D. Attitudes and motor skills
    E. All of the above

6. True or False: Before beginning a stakeholder consultation process, it is useful to think about who needs to be consulted, over what topics, and for what purpose.

7. When searching for health information via the Internet, a health education professional should be concerned about:
    A. The topic and potential benefits
    B. Synthesizing quality concerns
    C. Identifying criteria for evaluating online health information
    D. Critiquing the literature available online
    E. All of the above

8. True or False: Documenting consultation activities and their outcomes is not critical to effectively managing the stakeholder engagement process.

9. True or False: The first step in creating an effective presentation is to know your audience and understand its perspective.

10. True or False: PowerPoint slides, overhead projectors, blackboards, and whiteboards are "visual aids" and should be treated as such. They should be *visual*, focusing on graphics, illustrations, and plots rather than text.

11. Health education specialists and public health educators are dedicated to promoting healthy behaviors necessary to reduce and prevent disease, injury, and disability. Their specific responsibilities include:
    A. Assessing individual and community needs for health education
    B. Planning, implementing, and evaluating effective health education programs
    C. Coordinating the provision of health education services and acting as health education resources
    D. Communicating health education needs, concerns, and resources
    E. All of the above

12. True or False: To become a Certified Health Education Specialist, you must first receive a degree in health education, followed by an NCHEC certification.

Chapter 7: Communicate and Advocate for Health and Health Education

1. The "4 Ps of Marketing" are product, price, place, and _____.
    A. Prevention
    B. Promotion
    C. Progression
    D. Production

2. All of the following are types of advocacy except:
    A. Policy advocacy
    B. Grassroots advocacy
    C. Media advocacy
    D. Legislative advocacy

3. The format for writing a PSA includes the following guideline(s):
    A. The copy should be single spaced
    B. The bottom of the sheet should be marked with "###"
    C. The script should be split into two columns
    D. Both B and C

4. The Health Belief Model is an example of a _____.
    A. Cognitive theory
    B. Stage-step theory
    C. Scientific theory
    D. Paternalistic theory

5. All of the following are types of readability formulas except:
    A. Gunning Fog Index
    B. SMOG Readability Formula
    C. Fleming-Kirkland Grade Level Readability Score
    D. Frye Readability Formula

6. For readers with low literacy, educational materials should be developed at which grade level?
    A. 12th grade
    B. 10th grade
    C. 6th grade
    D. 3rd-5th grade

7. The acronym "GOTME" stands for:
    A. Goal, objective, timing, message, evaluation
    B. Goal, objective, target, market, evaluation
    C. Goal, objective, target, market, endpoint
    D. Goal, objective, target, message, evaluation

8. CUP research relates to which of the following area(s) of professional focus:
    A. Professional preparation
    B. Professional development
    C. Credentialing
    D. All of the above

9. Which of the following models are examples of stage-step theories:
    A. Transtheoretical Model
    B. Health Belief Model
    C. Perceived Behavioral Control Model
    D. Both A and B
    E. Both A and C

10. Health educators are prohibited from participating in _____.
    A. Direct lobbying
    B. Grassroots lobbying
    C. Electioneering
    D. None of the above

Test Your Knowledge—Answers

Chapter 1: Assess Needs, Assets, and Capacity for Health Education

1. True

2. E.

3. E.

4. D.

5. True

6. E.

7. True

8. False

9. True

10. F.

Chapter 2: Plan Health Education

1. C.
   "The community will participate in a safety-oriented bicycle ride" is an example of an appropriate learning objective. It is specific, measurable, and in terms of the learner. The first two choices are educator-centered, not learner-focused, and the school age child's understanding of proper hand-washing is not appropriate for the psychomotor domain (hand-washing technique), but instead for the cognitive domain.

2. A.
   Discussion is an appropriate teaching strategy for the cognitive domain of learning in addition to things like reading material, posters, and pictures. Role-playing is an effective strategy for the affective domain; demonstration, practice, and return demonstration are appropriate for the psychomotor domain of learning.

3. A.
   Primary prevention aims to prevent the occurrence of health problems, disease, and dysfunction before it occurs. Secondary prevention involves the early identification and treatment of specific health problems. Tertiary prevention aims to return the client to the highest possible level of functioning following the correction of a health problem.

4. D.

Repetition is one way that a teacher can help a learner with cognitive barriers. Other strategies for those with a cognitive deficit include clarification and re-clarification.

5. B.

Teaching methodologies must be consistent with the identified learning need, the domain, the level of the domain, and the learning objectives. Each learning need should be addressed with a separate learning objective and a correlated teaching methodology when the health educator has assessed multiple learning needs.

6. B.

The norming stage focuses on decision-making. The forming stage is the stage in which members are selected, goals are established, and orientation to the group occurs. The storming stage is included in some group process theories, as based on the fact that conflicts often occur in groups. The negotiation stage consists of task assignments and the assumption of roles, among other things.

7. D.

An example of a well-worded learning objective of the psychomotor domain is "After a CPR class, the student is able to perform CPR." The psychomotor domain is the doing domain, and the learning objective verbs for the psychomotor domain are *use* and *perform*.

8. C.

Sensory barriers to learning can be eliminated with the use of large print materials for the visually impaired. Other strategies include the use of Braille reading materials for the blind and speaking loudly for the auditory impaired.

9. A.

Sequencing content moves from the simple to the complex, from the non-threatening to the threatening, and from the known (or familiar) to the unknown (unfamiliar to the learner).

10. D.

All cultures have a unique vocabulary, slang, and/or terminology. Cultures share beliefs, values, practices, and communication patterns. Ethnicity is defined as a group of racially similar people of a similar origin, whereas culture is defined as a group of people who share values, ideals, and beliefs, regardless of their race and ethnicity. Bicultural people maintain more than one culture.

11. A.

Some of the ethical considerations for health educators include the presentation of current and scientifically sound principles and concepts, without bias or coercion. All humans are unique, and they have the right to make autonomous decisions without any coercion or undue pressure by others. Discrimination and reasonable accommodations for the disabled are legal, not ethical, concerns.

Chapter 3: Implement Health Education

1. C.

2. B.

3. A.

4. B.

5. B.

6. D.

7. A.

8. C.

9. A.

10. D.

Chapter 4: Conduct Evaluation and Research Related to Health Education

1. D.
   Quantitative research has a null hypothesis. This type of research is deductive. Conversely, qualitative research is inductive and contains no null hypothesis.

2. B.
   This review gives the researcher more information about the topic being studied and a deeper understanding of the research topic. It can also give the researcher ideas regarding concepts, possible research designs, and sampling techniques, among other things.

3. D.
   An example of a null hypothesis is, "Compliance rates will not increase after education." Quantitative research uses a null hypothesis. The null hypothesis is supported when the independent variable's manipulation does not statistically support any change in the dependent variable.

4. B.

A sample that is too small will lead to poor research results. A sufficient sample size is essential to sound research. Some suggest that a major research project should have 100 subjects; others say that fewer subjects are needed. Many studies use at least 30 subjects.

5. D.

The best data measurement tools are valid and reliable. Reliability reflects the measurement tool's ability to consistently measure the variable over time with the same results and among different data collectors (inter-rater reliability).

6. A.

Validity reflects the measurement tool's ability to actually measure what it is supposed to measure and nothing else.

7. B.

Likert Scales are the most commonly used scales. These scales measure how strongly a statement is agreed or disagreed to. They are relatively easy to construct, unlike Guttman Scales, and they work well with many statistical methods used in quantitative research.

8. C.

Measures of central tendency are the mean, mode, and median. The mean is the average of all of the values, or numbers, in the set of numbers; the mode is the most frequently occurring number, or score, in the set of numbers; and the median is the middle number in the set of numbers.

9. A.

When the result of the T-test is $p < .10$, it means that there is less than a 10% possibility that chance or accident has occurred. The results are primarily related to the research itself at about 90%. Likewise, $p < .05$ indicates that chance is less than 5%.

10. D.

Qualitative data is read thoroughly. It is then organized and examined closely for themes, patterns, and trends. The data is analyzed using inductive thinking and logic. This kind of research is used to discover an in-depth knowledge or description of the phenomenon being studied.

Chapter 5: Administer and Manage Health Education

1. E.

2. True

3. E.

4. True

5. MOA is a statement about a specific topic acknowledging cooperation between two or more parties and clarifying each party's roles and responsibilities. Compared to a standard contract, it is an attractive option and is much simpler to use. It helps both parties avoid distrust, potential insult, and possible resentment resulting from asking someone to sign a legal contract.

MOU stands for Memorandum of Understanding and MOA stands for Memorandum of Agreement. Two parties or partnerships use them for written agreements or a contract. Both agreements are developed between tribal and municipal governments to benefit a variety of environmental services and to maximize funding available for the community.

6. True

7. E.

8. E.

9. True

10. E.

Chapter 6: Serve as a Health Education Resource Person

1. F.

2. True

3. True

4. True

5. E.

6. True

7. E.

8. False

9. True

10. True

11. E.

12. True

Chapter 7: Communicate and Advocate for Health and Health Education

1. B.

2. B.
   Grassroots refers to a type of lobbying.

3. D.

4. A.

5. C.

6. D.

7. D.

8. D.

9. E.

10. D.
    Public charities are prohibited from electioneering.

CPSIA information can be obtained at www.ICGtesting.com
Printed in the USA
LVOW09s0231300916

506838LV00011B/162/P